THE PROFESSIONAL COMMITMENT: Issues and Ethics in Nursing

CARROLL A. QUINN, R.N., M.S.N.

Associate Professor of Nursing, Xavier University, Cincinnati, Ohio; Doctoral Candidate in Nursing, Indiana University, Indianapolis, Indiana

MICHAEL D. SMITH, Ph.D. (Phil.), M.H.A.

David C. Trew Fellow, Holy Cross Health System, South Bend, Indiana; Formerly, Assistant Professor of Philosophy, Xavier University, Cincinnati, Ohio

1987

W. B. SAUNDERS COMPANY

Philadelphia, London, Toronto, Sydney, Tokyo, Hong Kong

W. B. Saunders Company: West Washington Square
Philadelphia, PA 19105

Library of Congress Cataloging-in-Publication Data

Quinn, Carroll A.

The professional commitment.

1. Nursing ethics. I. Smith, Michael D., 1948– .
II. Title. [DNLM: 1. Ethics, Nursing. WY 85 Q7p]

RT85.Q56 1987 174′.24 86–27985

ISBN 0–7216–1098–6

Acquisition Editor: Dudley Kay
Production Manager: Frank Polizzano
Manuscript Editor: Edna Dick
Indexer: Sara Wilkerson

THE PROFESSIONAL COMMITMENT:
Issues and Ethics In Nursing ISBN: 0–7216–1098–6

Last digit is the print number: 9 8 7 6 5 4 3 2

PREFACE

The ideas for this book began to evolve as the authors were teaching what seemed to be quite different courses (nursing issues and bioethics) to the same group of registered nurses enrolled in a baccalaureate degree completion program. Through the informal dialogue typical among faculty who share a corridor, we quickly realized how many issues could not be fully discussed in either class without reference to content from the other. Student discussions about professional issues such as nurse-physician relationships, educational requirements, and economics often became lively discussions about conflicting loyalties to patients, colleagues, and employers. In recognizing the importance of collective activities for growth of the profession, students were also grappling with the effects of such activities on their responsibilities toward individual patients. Likewise, debates concerning traditional ethical issues such as the patient's right to know or to refuse treatment were peppered with these practicing nurses' personal experiences of the difficulties of respecting such rights in light of institutional constraints and nursing's perceived lack of autonomy within the health care system.

A review of available literature in the respective areas convinced us that, for the most part, clinical ethics and professional ethics in nursing were considered as separate sets of concerns. No one volume focused on the closely interwoven aspects of these issues. Thus began our venture into interdisciplinary dialogue and writing. Our goal in writing this volume was to address that gap in the literature and illustrate the artificiality of any separation of clinical ethics and professional issues, to emphasize that professional issues are ethical issues and that clinical ethical decisions are not made in a vacuum isolated from the broad professional concerns. Our venture has followed a long and circuitous route. It has been punctuated with lively debates and mutual mind-bending. We may have learned more about each other's disciplines than either of us cared to. But we became even more convinced of the appropriateness of our original intent as the volume developed. We did not intend to provide answers to the questions raised by our students and by each other along the route. What we hope we have done is provide you, the reader, with a slightly different and broader perspective on ethics and professional issues.

Acknowledgments

We are indebted to a number of people who have continued to support us during this project. We appreciate the support of our colleagues at Xavier University and Indiana University. Professors Lisa Newton of Fairfield

University and Mila Aroskar of the University of Minnesota both provided helpful suggestions at an early stage in the project's development. Lynn Hirt, Director of Nursing, and the nurse-managers of Margaret Mary Community Hospital provided regular feedback from practicing nurses.

We gratefully acknowledge the assistance of critical readers who provided numerous suggestions for improved organization and flow. Their insights and expertise have helped shape a more valuable, useful book for students and beginning practitioners.

Patricia Bennett, RN, MA
Anderson College
Anderson, Indiana

Margaret Benner, RN, Ph.D.
University of Delaware
Newark, Delaware

Pamela A. Miya, RN, MSN
University of Nebraska
Omaha, Nebraska

Gloria L. Rechlicz, RN, MSN Ed.
Marquette University
Milwaukee, Wisconsin

Caryle G. Wolahan, RN, Ed.D.
Felician College
Lodi, New Jersey

Donna Woodside, RN, Ed.D.
University of Cincinatti
Cincinatti, Ohio

Tillie Tanfani offered constant and invaluable assistance in library research. Our students, from whom the original ideas sprang, gave us continual feedback and insights that keep us true to our original intent. We are indebted to Dudley Kay of W. B. Saunders for his persistent yet gentle prodding. Finally, we wish to thank our families, who never wavered in their support, understanding, and tolerance of what sometimes must have seemed to them an endless venture.

CARROLL QUINN
MICHAEL SMITH

CONTENTS

Chapter One

PROFESSION AND ETHICS: AN INTRODUCTION

Nursing leaders have in recent years challenged the nursing community to examine professional and ethical issues. Increasingly sophisticated technology and increased awareness of nurses' responsibility for their own actions have led to greater consciousness of the ethical dilemmas that nurses face in practice. Educational curricula have responded to this new awareness, so that now it is difficult for the student nurse to avoid confronting some basic questions about clinical ethical issues. Questions about "pulling the plug," disobeying physicians' orders, disclosing patient information, obtaining informed consent, caring for defective newborns and other problems create ethical issues for nurses. Nurses in practice are flooded with invitations to hear speakers, to buy books, and to go to conferences that attempt to analyze these ethical problems from a nursing perspective. Somewhat less often, nurses function as ethicists or on ethics committees and institutional review boards in the institutions in which they practice.

Professional issues are commonly examined from sociological, economic, feministic, political, and historical points of view. Professional issues (such as nurse-physician relations, entry into practice, and economic concerns) are frequently discussed as if they were something separate from ethical issues. The result is that concerns about ethics seem to be limited to decisions made at the bedside. Ethical issues as nurses actually face them are in part a function of how professional issues are handled, but this important fact is easily overlooked in the current debates. Conversely, professional issues are often dealt with as if they were not at heart ethical issues. This dichotomy is artificial and harmful, for professional issues are ethical issues and ethical issues are professional issues. This important truth will be demonstrated through an examination of the nature of a profession, of ethics, and of how the two become interrelated in the context of professional practice. This interrelationship is shown through a discussion of matters usually considered professional issues rather than those normally understood to be part of clinical ethics.

Nursing's own claim to be a profession is the source of many of its major issues. Nursing, like a number of other occupational groups, is in a sort of nether region, a "gray area." Many of its members consider themselves professionals and act accordingly; others do not. Some members of society treat nurses as professionals and themselves as clients; others see nurses as unskilled but caring. There are major discrepancies in the social institutions that surround nursing: nurses are both autonomous professionals and dependent, semiskilled employees. It is difficult to classify nursing among the professions; but it is just as difficult to classify it with nonprofessional occupations. To the extent that the problem is merely one of terminology, it is not at all important to this volume's thesis. But professional life is a source of duties and values that are critical to daily practice. And the purpose of this volume is to explore the ethics of nursing as a true profession in the midst of the ambiguity that exists now.

Do not expect this work to provide the correct and definitive answers to the issues raised here. Although the building of a consensus is essential to a profession's collective efforts to solve its problems, some forms of consensus building are short-sighted. A consensus that ignores ambiguities and controversies is fragile and short-lived. Resolving professional issues requires that there be a consensus, but that it be achieved by minds used freely and openly, dealing with ambiguities and alternatives whenever they arise. The method of this work is to explore the issues from a variety of perspectives both to make relevant information stand out more clearly and to consider that information from the standpoint of a variety of ethical principles. Thus, this text attempts to formulate more clearly the issues themselves. It offers, in effect, a preamble to the resolution of professional issues, a basis for open thinking and debate.

This first chapter explores in general the meaning of the claim of nursing (or of any other occupation) to be a profession. Commitment plays a central role both in the concept of a profession and in its relation to ethics. Chapter 2 will develop more thoroughly the concept of ethics in a way that will make it useful for the examination of professional issues. Chapters 3 and 4 will begin the transition to more concrete issues, making use of the foundations provided earlier.

The remaining chapters will examine specific professional issues in more detail. In Chapter 10 guest author David Ozar reflects on the demands of professional obligation and the individual's right to have a private nonprofessional life. The problem of the professional, as he sees it, is how to integrate various commitments into a life as a whole person.

THE NATURE OF PROFESSIONS

Although the term "profession" is sometimes used in a purely descriptive way, a careful analysis of the nature of a profession will show that the idea of a profession carries with it some important ethical implications. To see this we will look first at a purely descriptive account of professions and then add to it the ethical implications. In everyday talk, we call some occupations "professions" but find it unusual to give that same name to other occupations. Ordinarily attorneys, architects, doctors, and members of the clergy are among those persons said to belong to the professions. Window washers, cab drivers, and short order cooks usually are not. One difference that stands out immediately is that persons in the professions enjoy higher social esteem, higher salaries, and more independence in their work. To leave the matter at that would be to fail to look below the surface.

The idea of a profession can be examined sociologically, which results in a descriptive account of the professions. The sociologist would first identify those occupations usually called professions and then determine what characteristics they have that nonprofessional occupations do not have. That list of characteristics is sometimes used as a way of classifying other occupations as either professions or nonprofessions. This is a descriptive approach and does not entitle us to draw any conclusions about what one's own occupation ought to be.

The heart and soul of professionalism escape those who limit their thinking about it to this descriptive model. In fact, professionalism must be viewed also from the perspective of those who choose to practice as professionals. Professionalism involves a personal promise and commitment and a parallel collective commitment by professionals as a social group. When these commitments are accepted and agreed to by society at large, they make sense of these various descriptive characteristics.

For nearly a century now, nursing has been dealing with the question of whether it, too, is a profession. Much of the discussion has followed the descriptive model, thus obscuring the ethical significance of the question. Some of the earliest discussions in nursing were reactions to a study done by the sociologist Abraham Flexner. In 1915 Flexner was asked to present an address on the professional status of social work. As his methodology, he proposed to first examine several occupations already most universally regarded as professions—law, medicine, and religion. In them he found a cluster of characteristics that he would use as a standard to examine social work: to the degree that social work displayed these same characteristics it, too, should be considered a profession. In his discussion, Flexner ventured an incidental judgment about the professional status of nursing: Nursing did not appear to be a profession because "...the responsibility of the trained nurse is neither original nor final" (Flexner, 1915, p. 581).

Many writers about nursing have accepted some variation of the criteria proposed by Flexner as well as his method. Although Flexner proposed a set of six characteristics of a profession, that number has been adjusted upward and downward by later authors. For present purposes, the idea of a profession is examined as a social institution that possesses rationally interrelated characteristics. The definition presented here distills four out of Flexner's six criteria and presents them in a rationally related way that describes the role that professions in fact have in our society. There may be additional characteristics, but the ones that follow are certainly a central part of the idea of a profession and will form the basis for subsequent discussions.

> THE PROFESSIONS ARE THOSE FORMS OF EMPLOYMENT THAT REQUIRE AN UNCOMMONLY COMPLEX KNOWLEDGE BASE, USED BY PERSONS COMMITTED TO THE DIRECT BENEFIT OF HUMAN BEINGS, WITH MINIMAL SOCIETAL CONTROL PLACED ON THEIR PRACTICE, AND ORGANIZED AMONG THEMSELVES TO ENSURE THAT THEY CONTINUE TO PROVIDE THOSE BENEFITS.

The professions have an uncommonly complex knowledge base. It is more than a coincidence that the number and variety of professions in society have increased with the greater sophistication of available technical knowledge. Architecture, engineering, and the practice of clinical psychology are examples of occupations that have become regarded as professions with the growth of technical knowledge. The growth of the professions in society results in part from the fact that we are increasingly dependent upon experts to serve us. It has become increasingly unreasonable to expect any one individual to master all the knowledge available and useful to serve personal health, legal affairs, financial affairs, and other important aspects of human welfare. The professions are those groups of experts on whom we depend to serve us with knowledge so complex that we cannot easily get it for ourselves. Thus, the professions usually require education within the university system, and often beyond the level of a four-year college degree. Members of the professions are usually engaged in research in order to ensure that their expertise is continuously upgraded. The education of new members of the professions is often supervised or controlled by those who are already practitioners.

The expert knowledge of the professional is used for the direct benefit of human beings. The professions are usually distinguished from those occupations that are openly self-serving. The man who earns a living for himself betting at the race track has an occupation, but that occupation is not called a profession, even if he has expert knowledge that enables him to consistently pick winners. Other occupations provide a service but do so only indirectly while attempting to make a profit. The individual who sells cars, for example, does serve those who need automobiles, but the most direct application of his knowledge is to making a profit. Some of the more complex accusations that someone has acted "unprofessionally" occur when it is judged that the pursuit of self-interest has dominated the attempt to benefit others. Such accusations typically come up when physicians are accused of ordering procedures that will benefit their own bank accounts rather than their patients, when teachers strike to gain pay increases, and in the other occasions when the client's needs lose out in a conflict with the professional's personal interests.

Minimal external control is placed on the practice of the professions. Although government usually places some restrictions on the ways in which the professions practice, these restrictions are ordinarily kept to a minimum. It is often unwise for nonexperts to make rules for experts, and society generally recognizes this. Even when government places some sort of constraint (such as professional licensure) on a profession, it is usually with the advice and consent of that profession. For example, state medical boards, which control medical licensing within individual states, usually have strong physician representation; bar associations perform similar functions for lawyers.

Because the amount of external control placed on an occupational group is a large-scale societal decision, it is possible for an occupational group not to be a profession simply because society has not offered it the opportunity to practice without a great amount of external control. Whether an occupation is a profession is, at least in part, a function of how society chooses to deal with that occupation. As frustrating as this may be for practitioners, their own efforts are not adequate to make their occupation a profession. How the rest of society deals with that occupation also determines whether it is a profession.

A profession is organized within itself for effective control of practice. A profession is not simply a collection of separate individuals, each of whom exemplifies the various characteristics of a profession. A profession consists also of a certain set of relations among those individuals, so that they are able to act as a group. Most of the recognized professions have organized into professional associations. Such associations typically provide opportunities for professional growth by sponsoring research, publication, and professional meetings. They provide a forum for debate of current issues facing a profession and sometimes recommend and influence legislation. They provide an internal control for the profession by developing codes of ethics and by censuring the unethical. Their control over licensure gives the profession some ability to remove the incompetent professional from practice. In effect, the collective efforts from within a profession to police its own ranks and to ensure continued competence substitute for societal control of the professions. Society delegates responsibility for the professions to the professions themselves.

The analysis of a profession presented here is in several respects idealized. Even the occupations that all would call professions do not always demonstrate these characteristics to perfection. Moreover, the professions are here portrayed as participants in a conscious and voluntary arrangement between themselves and the society they serve. Although there appears to be no single instance of a profession in which this is the case, emphasizing the voluntary "exchange" between society and its professions shows an important truth. The professions are social institutions that serve an important function in ensuring societal welfare, so a society might be very rational in according special freedoms to an occupational group that willingly serves that society with its unique expertise.

Over the years, writers about nursing have drawn a variety of conclusions about its professional status (Bixler and Bixler, 1945, 1959; Sleicher, 1981). Some writers have scored nursing on such criteria as the complexity of its knowledge base, the commitment and collective activities of its practitioners, and the extent to which society has imposed external controls on nursing. This volume will not add to the debate about whether nursing is already a profession. Its objective is instead to explore the meaning of professionalism in sufficient depth to see what professionalism demands of a nurse today. Without professional commitment, claims to professional status are empty noise. Although analysis of the descriptive characteristics of a profession may be illuminating, it is just as important to see nursing as it is faced by the individual who has made and understands the promise that amounts to professional commitment.

PROFESSION, COMMITMENT, AND ETHICS

In most of the professions, entry is marked by some public and ceremonial occasion in which the new professional makes a public proclamation of his or her intentions. Physicians, for example, have traditionally recited the Hippocratic Oath, and attorneys recite an oath when they are admitted to the bar. What is the significance of such an occasion? Pellegrino has summed up well what it is that the health care professional does on that occasion:

> The health professional makes a "profession." He or she "declares aloud" that he has special knowledge and skills, that he can heal, or help, and that he will do so in the patient's interest, not his own . . . . That is what entering a profession means—not simply becoming a member of a defined group with a common education, standards of performance, and a common ethic (Pellegrino, 1979).

Pellegrino's analysis expresses the very personal experience of entering a profession. The deeper meaning of profession is not out in the open for the observer to see: it is the experience of making a very personal decision to involve oneself in a system of roles that are socially defined. A professional commitment is somewhat different from private decisions. It is a public proclamation made to all potential users of the professional's services. Thus, it begins to involve other persons in a way that a purely private decision usually does not. In effect, the professional makes a *promise* to *society.*

Because the professions are socially defined, the content of that promise is not whatever the promisor wishes to make of it. Other members of society already know what a lawyer or physician should be, and they will hold accountable anyone who professes to be one. It is imperative for any profession examining its own ethics to understand what the content of its professional commitment is, not just in the minds of its own practitioners but in the minds of the other members of the society served by the profession. Thus, the promise embodied in professional commitment is public in two important ways—because it is made with the knowledge of the rest of society and because its content (*what* the profession promises) is a matter of public consent. One of the major ambiguities with which the professional nurse must contend is the discrepancy between the promise she wishes to make and societal disagreements about the nature and role of nursing.

When a decision is a purely private one, a change of mind is not always of concern to others. A decision to have the whitest shoes in the hospital can be altered when a trip to the beach seems more interesting than polishing shoes. But a promise made to others becomes a matter of ethics. A promise transforms the actions that follow from it. Although personal preference is often a good reason for doing or not doing something, once a promise has been made, the action in question can no longer be a matter of personal preference. The individual who has made the promise has a *duty* to act, and those to whom the promise is made have a *right* to what has been promised. There are certainly exceptions, but it is important to remember that the exceptions have to be justified. Such matters of rights and duties involve us necessarily in thinking about ethics.

Private decisions about what kind of employment to seek might well be matters of personal taste. But, as Pellegrino has noted, the difference between other forms of employment and the professions is that entry into a profession involves a personal and public promise to serve others with the special expertise that the profession can provide and that society legitimately expects it to provide. This is why professional issues are ethical issues: professional issues pertain directly to the profession's ability to live up to the promise it has made to society.

PROFESSIONAL COMMITMENT AND NURSING'S PROMISE

In 1893, when the graduating class of the Farrand School of Nursing in Detroit, Michigan, became the first group of nurses to recite the Nightingale pledge, it was likely that they did not realize the importance it would eventually acquire as a visible symbol of the nurse's professional commitment. For its formulators, it was to be a code of ethics, a set of guidelines for the new nurse to follow (Kalisch and Kalisch, 1986, p. 171). Large numbers of nurses practicing today have themselves recited the Nightingale pledge. However, the brevity of the pledge dictates that it be regarded as a *symbol* of the nurse's public promise to society rather than a literal expression of that promise. If nursing is a profession, perhaps we must look elsewhere to find what the nurse has promised.

What nurses have promised to do is probably not what they actually do. This may sometimes be the result of personal fault; when that is so, we say that the professional has engaged in *unprofessional behavior*. What is more common in the case of nurses is that constraints imposed by various features of the environment prevent them from practicing nursing in the way they have promised to practice. Moreover, there is great diversity in what nurses actually do, and much of what nurses do can be done by other health professions and ancillary personnel. One writer has gone so far as to claim that nursing itself is functionally redundant: "There is no job nurses perform that is not also performed by some other occupation" (Levi, 1980).

An accurate description of the commitment that nurses make must include a description of the actualities of practice. It must also include an account of the unrealized goals and ideals that nurses and the rest of society have for nursing. In 1980 the American Nurses' Association prepared a social policy statement that included a definition of nursing:

> Nursing is the diagnosis and treatment of human responses to actual or potential health problems (ANA, 1980).

This brief definition functions as a beginning point for describing the nursing commitment. In claiming that nursing deals with *human responses*, it emphasizes nursing's role in dealing not just with health problems but with living persons insofar as they are subject to the experience of health problems. The document cites a number of examples including self-care limitations, impaired function, pain, and self-image changes in relation to health status. The nurse deals not just with the conditions of the body but with problems of limitations and experiencing that are related to health status (Gadow, 1980; Curtin, 1979).

This first aspect of the nursing commitment is sometimes expressed with the distinction of cure from care. While physicians "cure," the role of the nurse is to provide "care" even when no cure is possible, desirable, or necessary. Certainly there is a difference between caring and curing. However, there is something dangerous in the presumption that physicians who cure without caring are doing what physicians ought to do. The social policy statement of the American Nurses' Association seems to be a more appropriate expression because it explains what nurses do while avoiding a territorial claim that unreasonably limits the physician's appropriate role.

Although nursing has long carried a public image of affective or emotive devotion to those persons who seek health care, professional nursing is more than this. The nurse *diagnoses* and *treats* responses. Diagnosing is a cognitive process: it requires knowledge and not just affection for one's patients. It demands an understanding of the processes of both the body and the mind and of human interactions. Professional nursing requires more than good will and affection; it requires sound knowledge. Nurses *treat* problems, so they must also be able to use knowledge in practice.

Some nurses are involved in functions other than the direct provision of care to patients. Some nurses teach other nurses; they conduct research; they organize and manage the activities of groups of nurses. Insofar as such activities are essential to the effective practice of nursing, they, too, are professional nursing activities. In fact, it will be argued in other parts of this volume that professional commitment requires that *all* nurses must be in some way involved in a broad spectrum of activities that make direct patient care more successful. What form that involvement should take is an ethical problem that the professional must continuously face.

Thus, the definition of nursing proposed in the American Nurses' Association statement is a useful beginning for analyzing the content of nursing's professional commitment, but it is not sufficient. Both nurses and the public whom they serve must understand what nursing has promised. This is an important difference between private decisions and the commitment that the professions make. A professional commitment is made loudly and publicly under conditions agreed upon by those making the promise and those to whom they are making it. There is an inescapable social dimension to the professions: they always involve a voluntary agreement between members of the profession and the society they serve. Clearly articulating the nature of a specific occupation is a prerequisite to its existence and recognition as a profession.

PROFESSIONAL CODES OF ETHICS

People who want their occupations to be regarded as professions sometimes point proudly to their group's code of ethics. In fact, when sociologists examine the standing of various occupations, they often look to see whether the group has collectively established for itself a code of ethics and now feels bound by it. A code of ethics of a profession is a set of principles to guide the individual practitioner. It ordinarily addresses some of the most common temptations that professionals might experience in the course of their practice, temptations to take advantage of the special power that their expertise gives them over clients.

Codes are important because professionals meet clients when they are especially vulnerable, i.e., when clients are dependent on the professional's expertise. Professional codes of ethics are more than just one more feather that the group wears to establish social recognition; they are, in fact, collective activities of the profession. The profession as a group establishes the code, pooling its wisdom and ethical good sense to create a set of guidelines that will address itself to the environment in which the profession is practiced. The profession *uses* its code to guide the instruction of new professionals and to sanction members who fail to honor it. As a result, the public whom the profession serves can rest assured that it can rely on the profession to provide the service to which it is committed, doing so within the limits of some basic ground rules. Having a code of ethics does not by itself make an occupation a profession. The code of ethics must be a collective enterprise by which the whole group feels bound and that is acceptable to society at large.

The first constitution of the American Nurses' Association (1897) proclaimed the need for a code of ethics, but it was not until 1950 that the association actually adopted one. From the first tentative discussions of a code to its most recent revision of the Interpretive Statements in 1985, the Code for Nurses has evolved. The code has consistently recognized nursing commitment, but it has gradually changed its claim about the persons to whom that commitment is made. Early versions stated that the nurse's most direct and primary obligation was to the physicians for whom she worked. Eventually there emerged a more developed view of the nurse as a true professional whose primary obligation is necessarily to her patients. In the 1976 version, all 11 principles of the code emphasize the primacy of duties to patients. In 1985, although the code itself remained unchanged, the Interpretive Statements emphasized even more explicitly the contract between nursing and the clients it serves.

The primacy of patients is most obvious in the principles that refer to *direct obligations* to them. Such direct obligations include protection of patient welfare and respect for confidentiality and privacy. *Indirect obligations* to patients involve actions that in the long run enable nurses to do what they have promised their patients. The code recognizes indirect obligations such as involvement in collective efforts to develop knowledge, to improve nursing standards and conditions of employment, and to improve health care on a societal scale. The code's recognition of indirect obligations to patients points to the fact that commitment to nursing care mandates both individual and collective efforts.

The code now relegates the nurse's relationship to the physician to an interpretative statement calling for "collaboration around the need of the client" (Code for Nurses, 1985, 11.4). This change is significant, for no longer can commitment to clients be subordinated to some higher duty. This, together with the recognition of indirect obligations, indicates a growing understanding of the relationship of a profession with its clients and its practice.

A profession's code of ethics is one of the most visible parts of the offer of commitment it makes to society. The offer should be one that the profession is prepared to live by, and it should be one that society is willing to accept. The Code for Nurses must remain a dynamic document, expressing both the conscience of nurses and nursing's relationship with society.

SUMMARY

To be a member of a profession is to make a personal commitment to provide a needed service to society using a special expertise. Moreover, to be a member of a profession is to be a member of a *group* of similarly expert and committed people, who work together to collectively honor their commitment. Groups of committed persons are a profession only when society recognizes their expertise and commitment and accords them a role consistent with professional standing. Social recognition depends, at least in part, on the group's ability to demonstrate to society the nature and necessity of its members' expertise and commitment. The evolution of the Code for Nurses and other recent documents indicates nursing's growing awareness of and ability to articulate the promise or commitment of professional nursing.

For Further Discussion

1. Discuss the relevance of the Nightingale pledge to contemporary nursing practice. Use the discussion of professions offered in this chapter to examine the adequacy of the Pledge as an explanation of nursing as a profession.

2. Review carefully the definition of nursing proposed in the American Nurses' Association's Social Policy Statement. Does it adequately express what nursing is and should be? Does it say it in a way that can be understood by the general public? Can you suggest improvements, from either your own thinking or reading?

Bibliography

American Nurses' Association (1980). A Social Policy Statement. Kansas City, Missouri: The Association.

American Nurses' Association (1985). Code for Nurses with Interpretive Statements. Kansas City, Missouri: The Association.

Bixler, G.K. and Bixler, R.W. (1945). The Professional Status of Nursing. American Journal of Nursing, 45:730.
Bixler, G.K. and Bixler, R.W. (1959). The Professional Status of Nursing. American Journal of Nursing, 59:1142.
Carroll, M.A. and Humphrey, R.A. (1979). Moral Problems in Nursing: Case Studies. Washington, D.C.: University Press of America.
Curtin, L. (1979). The Nurse as Advocate: A Philosophical Foundation for Nursing. Advances in Nursing Science, 1(3):1.
Flanagan, A. (1976). One Strong Voice: The Story of the American Nurses' Association. Kansas City, Missouri: American Nurses' Association.
Flexner, A. (1915). Is Social Work a Profession? Proceedings of the National Conference of Charities and Corrections. Chicago: Hildermann Printing Company.
Gadow, S. (1980). Existential Advocacy: Philosophical Foundation of Nursing. In Spicker, S. jand Gadow, S., editors (1980). Nursing: Images and Ideals. New York: Springer.
Kalisch, P.A. and Kalisch, B.J. (1986). The Advance of American Nursing. Boston: Little, Brown and Company.
Levi, M. (1980). Functional Redundancy and the Process of Professionalization: The Case of Registered Nurses in the United States. Journal of Health Politics, Policy and Law, 5(2):333.
Pellegrino, E.D. (1979). Toward a Reconstruction of Medical Morality: The Primacy of the Act of Profession and the Fact of Illness. Journal of Medicine and Philosophy, 4(1):32.
Sleicher, M.N. (1981) Nursing Is Not a Profession. Nursing and Health Care, (2):186.
Styles, M.M. (1982). On Nursing: Toward a New Endowment. St. Louis: C.V. Mosby Company.

Chapter Two

SOURCES FOR ETHICS

A professional code of ethics gives the practitioner access to some basic ethical rules in a way that can be readily applied to situations. But to assume that a profession's self-adopted code of ethics is the ultimate foundation for all the ethics the practitioner needs is to take a rather shortsighted ethical perspective. If a profession's code is not intended to conform to some more generally accepted ethics, it encounters at least two important difficulties (Veatch, 1979). First, there would be no reason for judging whether the professional group itself has acted either ethically or unethically in adopting a particular code. Second, the profession would have difficulty communicating its code of ethics and making it acceptable to the community that it intends to serve, because its ethics would become something akin to the arbitrary rules a private club establishes for itself.

The ethical rules or principles embodied in the profession's code of ethics are intended to reflect what people already believe about ethics in general and then to apply those beliefs to the current roles of that profession in society and to the kinds of ethical issues to which practitioners are typically exposed in those roles. Professionals may understand those roles better and foresee better than nonprofessionals the kinds of situations to which they are likely to be exposed. Ultimately, however, their professional code of ethics is derived from broader and more fundamental beliefs about ethics. Those more fundamental beliefs and the reasons for maintaining them are typically called *ethical theory*.

A code of ethics itself does not examine in great depth its own sources. A profession's code of ethics is intentionally brief and specific so as to encourage professionals to apply it readily. The purpose of the present chapter is to find the sources of ethics in order to reflect seriously and constructively on the issues of professional ethics.

An introduction to ethical theory must confront the matter of personal values. It would be unusual to find an adult who has no values. Most basically, values consist of attitudes toward everything to which a person is not indifferent. A person may attach either a positive or a negative value to something. Values are typically associated with the affective or emotional aspect of a person's life and are often viewed as determining how a person will act. Thus, it seems obvious that ethics and values are interrelated. Not everything that a person values is a matter of ethics. A person may value a trip to an art gallery for the beauty of the sculpture that is there, a chocolate eclair (and perhaps the recipe for it), or a pun that would make most other people groan. Such values are often considered *matters of personal taste.* In matters of taste there is no reason for agreeing or disagreeing with another's choice. A Latin proverb states that *"De gustibus non est disputandum";* matters of taste are not worthy of debate.

Matters of ethics differ from matters of taste. Ethical issues do seem to be worthy of debate, and it does seem to be important to have some reasons for the values that one upholds. Some of the more controversial questions of ethics arise when one attempts to differentiate between values that are matters of personal taste and those that are matters of ethics.

Efforts to engage in *values clarification* do not address the important difference between matters of taste and ethical values. Values clarification uses structured exercises to identify what one really values and how those values result in action (Steele and Harmon, 1979). It is useful as a process of taking inventory of the kinds of things that one in fact values. But values clarification itself does not distinguish between the values that one holds as a matter of ethics and those that are not ethical values. Therefore, clearer understanding of ethics itself is necessary. Attention to four important characteristics of ethics will help distinguish between those values that are ethical and those that are not.

1. Ethics consists of values that a person uses as rules or principles to make decisions. A rule or principle for action is a general statement of what to do and can be applicable to a number of similar cases. To the extent that a value is a person's ethical value, that person uses it to deal with similar situations similarly. Thus, ethics has a *consistency* to it that is not necessarily found in all of a person's other values (Hare, 1952).

2. Ethical values are the values that a person thinks ought to take priority over other values when making decisions. Values often begin to conflict with one another when a person acts on them. Ethical values are the ones that a person believes ought to override all other values in life and serve as the basis for decisions in such conflict situations. Persons sometimes act on values that are different from the ones that they think ought to

override other ones; they do not always adhere to their own ethics. Therefore, we cannot look simply to what a person actually does in order to know what that person thinks is ethical.

3. A personal ethic consists to some extent in the way in which other persons are valued. There is tremendous variation in the ways different ethical theories deal with the problem of how to treat other persons. However, if there is not some value attached to other persons (to their welfare or their liberty, for example), those values would not really form an ethic.

4. An ethic consists of those values (and principles based on them) that have been given thoughtful consideration. To apply a certain group of principles consistently throughout one's life and to give those values top priority is a major life commitment. It is therefore natural to examine them carefully to determine which values should be given such a status and why this should be so.

The project of finding some values out of which to develop a personal ethic is highly personal, and there are few initial rules to guide one in the endeavor. Those who undertake it can benefit from the several thousand years of experience of others who have produced some of the most comprehensive and thoroughly criticized proposals for a personal ethic. This chapter will examine some of the most enduring proposals. The final section of this chapter will show how development of a personal ethic (which is sometimes called a personal morality) is a prerequisite to the development of a professional ethic.

UTILITARIANISM: A CONSEQUENTIALIST APPROACH TO ETHICS

One useful first step in developing a personal ethic is to identify the kinds of feelings one already has about good and bad, right and wrong. The utilitarian finds a single basic feeling at the heart of all decision-making and develops the utilitarian principle out of that feeling. In order to see clearly the utilitarian point of view, consider the following three situations:

SITUATION 1. An underground gas explosion suddenly sends a mass of people to the emergency room. The facilities are inadequate to give prompt care to everyone who comes in. The hospital triage team moves swiftly from person to person, determining whether immmediate care is essential. Divisions are drawn between those who would not survive even with care, those who will survive without it, and those for whom immediate care will make a crucial difference.

SITUATION 2. Denise R. has recently read about problems of starvation in certain African countries and has decided to do something to help. In today's mail she received solicitations from two different relief agencies. The first one uses 93 per cent of all donations for direct relief, reserving 7 per cent for administrative costs. The second agency uses 84 per cent for aid, keeping 16 per cent to cover costs. Denise sends a check to the first agency.

SITUATION 3. The staff nurse on a medical surgical unit is working the 11 to 7 shift. The unit is short-staffed tonight. She has to set priorities, deciding who should get medication first, whether she can afford a few extra minutes to talk with one restless patient, how often to turn another patient, and so forth. In order to make these decisions in an orderly way, she adopts as her operating motto for the evening, "Who needs it worst gets it first."

In each of these cases, the decision-maker looked primarily to the results of actions, to what would be accomplished by them, in order to determine what to do. Theories that approach ethics in this way can be called *consequentialist* theories. Consequentialist theories of ethics all have in common their emphasis on results, but they do not always agree on what should be considered ethically important concerning these results. Utilitarianism is one form of consequentialist ethics.

In the cases just cited the decision-makers chose to do what would provide the greatest benefit, not just for themselves but for as many people as possible. They may not have done this as a matter of principle; perhaps it just felt comfortable and natural to do the most good possible. The utilitarian respects that feeling and proposes that it be made into a principle or rule to apply to all cases in which a decision must be made. This principle is commonly called the *principle of utility* (Mill, 1863).

Utilitarianism is the view that the principle of utility should be the foundation for a personal ethic. It is the belief that doing what is morally good *always* consists of surveying the possible courses of action open to us, determining their effects on the welfare of *everyone* who will be affected by them, and then choosing the course of action that will do the most good coupled with the least harm for as many people as possible. The consequences of our actions are of paramount importance in this way of looking at ethics. No action is in itself either good or bad. The only thing that makes an action good or bad is the consequences that are likely to result from it.

The attempt to capture this feeling of concern for everyone and express it as a moral principle leads to the discovery of an ambiguity in the feeling: trying to bring about good consequences is futile without some view of what makes a consequence good or bad. One early utilitarian, Jeremy Bentham, proposed that pleasure is the only good thing and pain the only bad (Bentham, 1789). According to him, there is no such thing as an inherently evil pleasure. Actions become evil only when they have consequences that are painful. This particular approach to utilitarianism is *hedonistic* utilitarianism.

John Stuart Mill made a somewhat different claim about good and bad consequences in his effort to reflect more closely the ordinary person's views on the matter (Mill, 1863). He thought that the term "pleasure" was a little too vague to tell us much. The pleasure of learning, the pleasure of reading a good mystery novel, the pleasure of sex, the warm feeling we get from an act of friendship, the relief of having survived a serious illness, and the psychopath's pleasure at a torture-murder are all called "pleasure." Mill insisted that pleasures are different from each other and that these differences are important for developing an ethic. There are higher and lower pleasures, according to Mill, and to find out which is which we must discover the actual preferences of the most widely experienced among us. Mill's form of utilitarianism is distinctive because of its emphasis on the varieties of good consequences.

A third alternative is to refrain from identifying what specific aspect of consequences make them good or bad and to concentrate instead on the *preferences* of those who will be affected by the act. This form of utilitarianism would hold that consequences are good insofar as people prefer them over other consequences (Beauchamp and Childress, 1983, p. 23). Economists find this form of utilitarianism particularly attractive because there is often a close relationship between what people prefer and what they consume, and between how much they prefer something and what they are willing to pay.

All these various formulations of the utilitarian ethics have a common feature: ethics is somehow based on what consequences people actually want from their actions. This explains the appeal of utilitarianism. One twentieth century writer has shown why this makes utilitarianism appear to be a very reasonable personal ethic:

> No ethical first principle can be strictly proved. All that one can do is to present considerations that will lead honest and reasonable people to accept such a principle. . . . Each person desires his own happiness. Therefore, a first principle that makes happiness good will prove acceptable to honest men when they consider it (Hall, 1968).

According to the utilitarian view of life, the ultimate judge of what people *should* want from life is what well-informed and honest people *actually* want. There is no higher appeal in ethics, according to this view.

Not everyone agrees that utilitarianism satisfactorily explains feelings about right and wrong. It is sometimes claimed that a utilitarian morality would require us to believe things about ethics that, in all honesty, we do not actually believe. For example, it might require that we break a promise or take a life whenever we can do more good than by keeping the promise or respecting that life. It might require harvesting healthy organs from the elderly in order to support the young, if they have a greater potential for future happiness. Or it might require that I not pay back money that I owe, if I have found a better use for it.

The form of utilitarianism to which such criticisms are usually addressed is called *act utilitarianism*. The act utilitarian holds that the consequences of each specific act determine whether that act is good or bad. Another form of utilitarianism tries to deal with such criticism. *Rule utilitarianism* holds that we should not judge how much our actions individually will affect human welfare. Instead, we should ask what the consequences would be if everyone acted in the way that I propose to act. To a rule utilitarian, killing an innocent party might be morally wrong even if in this particular situation one can produce greater welfare by doing so. In the long run, human welfare might be better served if we all observed a rule of not killing innocent people. A similar statement might be made about keeping promises. Although one can sometimes do more good by breaking a promise or commitment than by keeping it, the long-range interest of humanity might be better served if everyone adopted a rule that promises ought always to be kept. It should be noted that, in the long run, even the rule utilitarian holds that *consequences* determine the ethics of action. Thus, there is still a basic disagreement between utilitarians and their critics.

As a system of ethics utilitarianism has much to recommend it: concern for human welfare and concern for the consequences of our actions do both seem to be close to the heart of morality. Whether they are the *only* things that should be at the heart of ethics is another matter. We will look at some other views that disagree with utilitarianism on this point.

DUTY-BASED ETHICS (DEONTOLOGY)

A group of alternative views of ethics takes issue with the utilitarian claim that results or consequences are the only element ultimately important in ethics. Consider the administration of a placebo to a patient complaining of chronic pain but in danger of becoming drug-dependent. The effective use of a placebo requires that the patient believe he is receiving active medication. Nurses, in their hospital duties, are sometimes called upon to help create the deception that makes a placebo effective (Bok, 1974; Brody, 1977).

A utilitarian would likely consider consequences such as the dangers of drug dependency, the value of pain relief, and the possibility of harm caused by a loss of trust should the deception be discovered. A rule-utilitarian, on the other hand, would seek to determine what the consequences would be if it became a general rule or policy to give or refuse to give placebos in all similar cases. Both the rule-utilitarian and the act-utilitarian believe that in some way the consequences of giving a placebo wholly determine whether it is right or wrong.

Some who disagree with utilitarianism believe that there is something inherently wrong with acts of deception regardless of consequences. Such critics argue that utilitarians account for only one of the many intuitive feelings about right and wrong and have elevated it to the status of a supreme principle. Acts such as the direct termination of human life, mandatory genetic screening, and so forth, should not be evaluated exclusively by the results they are likely to yield. Killing other people or forcing them to undergo tests may be ethically wrong even if doing so on specific occasions or as a general rule produces beneficial results.

A view of ethics built upon the belief that duty is as fundamentally important as good consequences is called a *deontology*. The common thread running through various forms of deontological ethics is that they all claim that ethics is not simply a matter of producing good consequences—that we have an ethical duty or obligation to do or to avoid doing some things regardless of the consequences. Deontologists differ among themselves about *which* ethical principles should determine a person's duties or obligations. Two different deontological thinkers, Immanuel Kant and W. D. Ross, are examined here.

Kant and the Categorical Imperative

Immanuel Kant believed that the basic problem of ethics is what it takes to be a person of good will. When he wrote his first little treatise on ethics in the late 1700's, he began by claiming that "nothing . . . could be called good without qualification except a good will" (Kant, 1785, First Section). He quickly followed that up with the common-sense reminder that whether one is a person of good will should not be judged by accomplishments.

The term *will* refers to the ability to take conscious control over one's own action. To choose to work in a hospital is often done of one's own will. To trip and spill some medication without intending to is usually not a willful action. Kant believed that human beings are capable of willing in a special way because of their capacity to be rational. Nonrational animals act instinctively without formulating a plan for action. Humans, instead, routinely develop general policies and then apply them to specific situations to formulate a course of action. As an example, consider a nurse who verifies with the attending physician a medication order for a patient whose condition has changed since the order was written. In deciding to verify the order, Kant would claim that the nurse had adopted a general policy (to verify all orders for treatments that appear not to be in the patient's best interest). Using the general principle, the nurse arrives at a specific course of action (to call Dr. Jones before administering digoxin 0.25 mg to Mrs. Brown, whose pulse is 52). Applying general principles to specific situations is the way in which human beings ordinarily make decisions. Kant calls it "rational will," because it is an exercise of both the capacity to reason and to will at the same time.

The basic problem of ethics, according to Kant, is whether there are some policies or principles best suited to a rational will. Persons of good will use their will in the most rational way possible. Kant argues that the most rational use of the will would lead us to adopt only those policies that could at the same time be willed to be a universal law. He proposes as a test to always ask whether the policies or principles that I adopt for myself are ones that I can consistently recommend that every other rational being also adopt. Kant called this test the *Categorical Imperative.*

Philosophers have argued for almost two centuries about what Kant meant by this and about what kind of lifestyle would result from such a view of personal ethics. Kant himself offers the example of breaking promises. Sometimes more good can be done by breaking a promise than by keeping it. For a rational being to break the promise would involve having adopted a general policy of breaking promises whenever doing so can bring about more good than keeping them. A person of good will (a person with a fully *rational will)* would subject this policy to a test: Could it become a policy for everyone to follow?

Kant responds that, if everyone felt free to break promises whenever something could be gained by doing so, there could no longer be any such things as promises. Part of the very definition of a promise includes the obligation or duty to do what is promised. If, as a matter of policy, we all agree that there is no such duty, we have in essence claimed that there is no such thing as promising. So, Kant concludes, it is irrational to claim to make a promise when you believe at the same time that you are not obligated to keep the promise. The policy of breaking promises in order to do good simply cannot satisfy the test that Kant claims a person of good will would use.

It is important to see that Kant does not claim that breaking promises is wrong because of the consequences that would follow if everyone did so. That would be a rule-utilitarian argument. Kant, instead, claims that we cannot even make sense out of the concept of promising without the recognition that promises entail duties to keep promises. Thus, we cannot rationally adopt a policy of breaking promises on the basis of good consequences.

Kant offers another way of testing policies for action to make sure that they are consistent with our status as rational beings. The Categorical Imperative requires that we recognize that each individual is a rational, willful being living in community with other rational, willful beings. So, if we treat all persons as beings with their own rational will rather than as objects to use for our own purposes, we are being of good will. This formulation of the Categorical Imperative is remarkably close to the Golden Rule but is arrived at without direct appeal to its traditional religious context.

In this second formulation we can see better the kinds of duties that the Categorical Imperative would place in a personal ethic and in a professional code of ethics. To hasten the death of a dying man in order to make use of his organs for transplant is to use him for our goals rather than to consider him as a rational being with a will of his own. We are treating him as a means toward some other good rather than as a rational, willful person (Ramsey, 1970). Similarly, using a patient for research that will not benefit him directly or giving a patient's health records to some third party for commercial use might be very obvious violations of the principle of treating persons as ends rather than just as means. Kant's categorical imperative, when seen under this second description, turns out to be a fundamentally important moral principle. In it Kant has found a way of combining his beliefs that rationality is good and that we should treat all persons in ways that respect their humanity. Feelings of duty that arise on occasions such as the placebo case cannot be erased by doing as much good as possible. They must be accounted for in our personal ethic. Kant was convinced that the Categorical Imperative could account for these feelings, because it began with fidelity to our nature as beings with rational wills.

Ross and the Ethical Duties of Human Relationships

W. D. Ross, a twentieth century deontologist, agrees with Kant that the effort to produce good results cannot by itself constitute a completely ethical life (Ross, 1930). Utilitarians, he claims, seem to assume that the only important feature of a relationship with other people is that they can be "possible beneficiaries of my action." In fact, other people can be much more than this: they can be spouses, debtors, creditors, friends, or dependents. All such relationships bring with them new duties owed to those people with whom one is interrelated. Ross believes that the basic ways in which human beings are interrelated are understandable only when the duties and obligations in those relationships are understood. Duties are not rules of conduct imposed on our relations with others from the exterior. Instead, they are part of our own understanding of a relationship that we enter. The duties define the particular relationship.

Human beings first become aware of their duties in specific relationships on specific occasions. One who has the ability to do good or prevent harm to another on some specific occasion knows almost intuitively that it is a duty to do so. A person who has made a promise to someone has established a different sort of relationship, one that now includes a duty to do what was promised. A person who has borrowed money thinks naturally that the relationship now includes a duty to pay back that money. All this is thought without any highly abstract philosophical reasoning. Instead, it is part and parcel of our natural everyday perceptions of the situations and relationships in which we exist.

Eventually, with experience of enough individual relationships, we begin to make more general judgments about duties or obligations in relationships. We begin to think, for example, that we have a duty to help others *whenever* we are able to do so (a duty of *beneficence*) and a duty to avoid harming others when we can (a duty of *nonmaleficence*). In fact, the utilitarian has accounted for these two duties. In similar manner, we become aware that there are general duties to keep promises and remain faithful and true in other ways (duties of *fidelity*), duties to repay the beneficence of others (duties of *gratitude*), and so forth. The utilitarian has not accounted adequately for these other facets of human relationships and thus does not give them their proper place in ethics, according to Ross.

In any one situation, there may appear to be several such duties. Duties may conflict with each other, so that it is not always possible to act on all of them. There can be conflicts between keeping a promise of confidentiality to one person and doing good for another (e.g., in the reporting of contagious diseases). Similarly, acting beneficently toward one person can result in acting maleficently toward another (e.g., by hastening the death of one person in order to supply a donor organ for another). The general duties that we would usually call our ethical duties or obligations are only *prima facie* duties; they appear at first to be our duties.

Relationships make conflicting demands. The various roles one takes on in life do not always fit together in an absolutely orderly pattern. Ross has pointed out that the demands of roles and relationships form a foundation for ethics, but he also says that there is no obvious answer about what to do when the duties of various relationships begin to conflict. He acknowledges that there can be no cookbook approach to resolving such conflicts. The best resource for the resolution of conflicting ethical demands is careful personal reflection on the acts that we feel called upon to perform because of the relationships we are in.

Ross has proposed a different way of understanding the most fundamental problems of ethics: ethics involves understanding the legitimate demands ("duties") that define roles and relationships. Ethics is not primarily the search for some ultimate standard by which to assess our actions. Nor is it encapsulated in some thought process that may be followed step by step to guarantee an ethical conclusion. Instead, it is a matter of understanding the relationships in which we actually find ourselves. If ethics begins with apprehending and defining our specific interpersonal relationships, it is possible that ethics will be very dependent on the culture in which we live our own lives, for culture structures human roles and relationships. (Ross has sometimes been criticized for assuming in his writings that the ethical person will be the same sort of well-bred English gentleman that he himself was.)

In reflecting on the nature of the professions and how they give rise to ethical obligations, one sees better the value of Ross's insight. The professions are special sorts of relations that exist among people in our society. Reflecting on how an occupational group is related to the rest of society is essential to understanding the duties of professional ethics and the issues that it deals with. The examination of nursing in this volume is ıeally an attempt to examine more fully nursing's relationships with the rest of society and to uncover and reflect upon the duties that define that relationship.

Duties and Rights

A deontological ethic (one built upon the idea of *duties* as the primary feature of ethics) leads into another feature of everyday morality of which we must take account—the matter of *rights.* The belief that there are ethical duties considers only one end of relationships. Relationships commonly involve an identifiable person to whom the duty is owed. That person is said to have a *right* to what another has a duty to do or provide. The belief that people have a right is the belief that they are legitimately entitled to something, that it is owed to them. It is the "other half" of the belief that people have duties to others (Feinberg, 1970; Dworkin, 1977).

Kant's example of promise-keeping serves well to show how duties and rights can be interrelated. To make a promise is to put oneself under a new duty, to do what one has promised to do. The person to whom a promise is made not only *expects* but *deserves* to have the promise kept. We express this deservingness by saying that this person now has a *right* to what was promised.

Adding the idea of rights to moral and ethical thinking expands the understanding of ethics to include a logically intertwined system of duties to act in certain ways and rights to be treated in certain ways. This is especially important in the ethics of health care. Professional ethics is not just a list of rules that make up the professional's ethical duties; it must include also a recognition of the rights of those whom professionals serve. Exactly what those rights are is a matter of ongoing dialogue. The statement of the American Hospital Association in the Appendix is one example of an effort to identify key rights within the health care setting.

There is a remarkable similarity between the concepts used in ethics and those used in legal thinking. We think and speak of *legal* rights and *legal* duties just as we do of ethical rights and duties. But it is important to realize that there can be important differences between legal thinking and ethical thinking. To have a moral right to something is not the same as to have a legal right to it. Moral rights do not always have the power of law to back them up. This may be due to imperfections in the legal system, but it may also be due to the undesirability of legally enforcing every part of our ethics. As a matter of fact, many of the rights listed in the American Hospital Association statement and other similar statements are also legally enforceable. But they could still be moral rights even if they did not have the power of the law to back them up.

This theoretical distinction between having a moral right and having a right enforceable by law is important in practice. First, the distinction points to a deeper ethical significance behind the legal protocol that professionals must follow in their practice. Legal requirements such as informed consent require of the nurse who signs them as a witness only an acknowledgment that the patient has been viewed putting his signature on the form. Informed consent is also a protection of the patient's autonomy and has important ethical implications; it is a way of offering patients basic human respect, a sort of respect to which they have a moral right regardless of the law.

Second, health care professionals need to take a special long-range interest in the ethical dimensions of legislation affecting their practice. They must be able to have a perspective on the law other than the perspective of the law itself in order to evaluate those changes. An ethical perspective on legislative matters provides a basis for evaluating law and seeking changes when necessary. Without such a perspective, professionals might find themselves having to practice in situations in which there is no legal support for their efforts to practice ethically.

In summary, a deontological understanding of ethics begins with the idea of morality as consisting of duties and not just of efforts to bring about the best possible results. It can reasonably be extended to include the related concept of rights. Exactly what these duties and rights are is a matter still debatable. We have seen how two thinkers in this tradition would go about establishing what our duties are.

THE NATURAL LAW TRADITION AND ETHICS AS VIRTUE

Utilitarianism and most deontological views of ethics have one important thing in common: they begin from the assumption that ethics is primarily a way of making decisions about individual actions or patterns of action. It is possible to begin ethics with a different assumption: that the most basic questions in ethics are about *what a person should be.* With such a view, how one acts in specific situations is important only because it demonstrates some more permanent feature of the person, i.e., that person's *character,* which is often described by attributing *virtues* to the person. Historically, that viewpoint has developed together with the *natural law* tradition in ethics. Although they can be considered separately, we shall deal with both the natural law tradition and the virtue tradition (sometimes called "aretaic") together.

What should a person be? Is there such a thing as real human growth and maturity beyond purely physical maturation? The same question is more commonly asked introspectively: are there changes I can make in myself that would make me a better person? People deal often with such questions even without realizing that they are doing so. Parents, to give just one example, must judge what developmental changes are desirable for their children: is it more important to be self-sufficient or cooperative, intellectual or emotive, a good fighter or nonviolent, and so forth? Those responsible for the education of society's youth face the same kind of questions because of their professional relationship to their students. Professionals as well often face questions about qualities worth developing that are not easily reducible to questions about which act is the right one. Both individual professionals and those responsible for educating and licensing members of the profession deal with such questions.

By focusing ethical thinking only on actions, one begins to think of a human life as nothing more than a set of separate, independent events. This is an unrealistically limited description of how people actually think of themselves existing in the world. In fact, persons think of themselves as having (or lacking) certain qualities by which they define themselves over an extended period of time. They think of themselves with inherent potential that can be either developed or neglected. An approach to living can be expressed adequately only in the whole direction of a person's life and not in individual actions viewed in isolation from one another. The tradition in ethics that considers virtue paramount sees the importance of such a holistic approach to ethics, and it is supported by traditional views concerning a natural law.

How should one decide what would be a better life for a person, what personal qualities to develop and nurture over time? Simply saying that it is "up to the individual" is not a sufficient answer. Such a response correctly identifies *who* must face the problem, but it says nothing about *how* reasonable human beings might begin to solve the problem they face. Individuals sometimes wonder whether there is any *reason* for thinking that one way of developing a life would be inherently better than some other.

In dealing with this question, some thinkers have proposed that there is a *natural law* of human existence, a kind of plan or basic orderliness, a purpose, to life. The rhythmic progression of the seasons, the harmonic movements of the stars and planets, and the functionality of the various organs of the human body have all, at one time or another, been taken as evidence of a basic plan to the universe itself. Perhaps a plan for human development is part of this basic orderliness of the universe. If there is such a plan, the most fundamental question of ethics concerns humanity's proper place in the grand scheme of the universe. Or perhaps there is a developmental plan for human growth even if the larger universe has none. Both of these two possibilities express what is meant by a *natural law* that is the source of ethics.

The natural law view of ethics has been attractive to some theistic thinkers who believe that there is a basic plan for the universe and objectively valid goals for human life within it. This fits handily with the belief that there is a Planner and Creator. In fact, natural law theory became the basis for much of Roman Catholic moral theology, which has produced copious literature on health care ethics in the twentieth century. Much of the theological work in ethics within this tradition has been built upon the work of Thomas Aquinas. Within this particular Christian view of the natural law, our attempts to make ourselves more fully human are at the same time a form of respect for God's plan for us.

Other thinkers in the natural law tradition have not built their beliefs about ethics on a belief in God. As early as 400 B.C. Aristotle spoke of the development of our rational abilities as a means of controlling our irrational impulses. In developing our capacities for conscious choice rather than instinctual behavior, Aristotle believed that there is a better chance of achieving the basic human goods that make a human life a happy one, goods such as virtue, health, and friendship (aided, ideally, by a modicum of wealth).

One of the most valuable contributions of the natural law tradition in ethics has been its emphasis on the importance of developing *personal character* as the focal point of ethics. A person of good character is the kind of person who habitually wants to do what is right, almost as a matter of second nature. This second nature can be analyzed into different areas of habitual judgment and action, each of which is called a *virtue*. Among the virtues commonly judged to be essential to the development of character in this ethical tradition are courage, temperance, truthfulness, and modesty. These are seen not only as resulting in particular actions but as indicating and forming the kind of person one is.

In the twentieth century, much of what was formerly regarded as ethics in this natural law tradition has reappeared in psychological thinking. By identifying the characteristics of a fully mature adult person and using those characteristics as the goals of psychotherapy, clinical psychologists have continued the tradition of specifying proper goals for human existence. Carl Rogers in *On Becoming a Person*, for example, claims that we become a person to the extent that we become open to new experience (Rogers, 1961). And Eric Fromm has proposed that the "aim of man's life is...the unfolding of his powers according to the laws of his nature." While Fromm recognizes the universal aspect of ethics, he has the awareness of individual differences that modern psychology has given us:

> While sharing the core of human qualities with all members of his species, he differs by his particular blending of character, temperament, talents, dispositions. . . . He can affirm his potentialities only by realizing his individuality (Fromm, 1947).

When people have begun examining the question of optimal states for human existence, they have sometimes varied in their answers. Still, the core question recurs both throughout the individual's life and throughout the history of ethics: what should a person strive to become?

THE RELIGIOUS DIMENSION

Beliefs about what is ethical are often bound up together with religious beliefs. People who believe that there is a being who created and rules the universe and who decides the ultimate destiny of human beings will naturally consider these beliefs in deciding what is most important to do on a day-to-day basis. It would be impossible (and unfair) to present here one particular way of believing about religion's relationship to ethics as *the* religious approach to ethics; there is much diversity in this relationship and also in ethical beliefs even among those who share common religious beliefs. Western religious ethics can be broadly characterized by focusing on two differing orientations, one emphasizing obedience and the other emphasizing love.

To some religious believers, obedience to the commands of God is the heart of ethics. Recognition of the omnipotence of God and of our subjection to God requires acknowledgment of our proper place in the scheme of things, namely obedience to God's command. Those who espouse this kind of ethics often look to Scripture for the content of these commands. Some also believe that God continues to speak to human beings through prayer. But there is disagreement about where and how God communicates commands. Even among groups who agree, there can still be a problem in applying general commands (such as the Ten Commandments) to particular situations. Ethical issues in contemporary health care may present especially difficult problems if God's commands are revealed only in scriptures or traditions formed long before the development of contemporary technology and social institutions such as the professions.

Another religious ethical tradition has been built on the theme of *agape*, or unconditional love. The focus of ethical thinking, according to this view, should be relationships with others, with God's own love for us proposed as a perfect relationship to imitate. The agapaic ethic can be found in the Christian tradition:

> Love the Lord your God with all your heart and with all your soul and with all your mind and with all your strength. The second is this: "Love your neighbor as yourself." There is no commandment greater than these (Mark 12:30-31).
>
> For God so loved the world that he gave his only begotten Son... (John 3:16).

Situation Ethics. Situation ethics disputes the possibility of building principles of ethics on the basis of love and holds that all one can ever do is act in each unique situation as lovingly as possible (Fletcher, 1966). But other agapaic thinkers argue that it is both possible and important to develop general ethical principles within a context of ultimate love (Niebuhr, 1935).

Religious ethics is not completely different from the other traditions of ethical theory discussed here. A religious ethic that emphasizes strict adherence to the scriptural Ten Commandments, for example, is another sort of deontological ethics. And an ethic that emphasizes the central role of love and loving relationships might parallel in many ways the utilitarian aim of doing as much good for as many people as possible. Alternatively the Golden Rule, which is a frequent expression of the Christian ethic of love, sounds very similar to Kant's Categorical Imperative, especially in the formulation that claims that we should treat all humans as ends having their own purposes rather than simply as means. Perhaps the importance of a religious ethic is greatest in the way in which it relates questions about right and wrong to other basic questions and answers about the nature and purpose of human existence.

CONCLUSION

A list of ethical theories such as the one presented here might appear to be like a cookbook from which one can choose a menu according to personal tastes. But ethics is an effort to act reasonably, i.e., in a way consistent with fundamental beliefs about human nature, the world that humans exist in, and their relationship to whatever supernatural reality there might be. Professional ethics and the codes in which it is embodied is an attempt to apply a more general view of ethics to the specific situation of the profession. Thus, the understanding of professional ethics requires an understanding of the profession itself as well as of the deeper foundations of ethics. Professional ethics without this deeper foundation is little more than a set of arbitrary rules, much like the rules of etiquette that gain their power from sheer custom.

It is possible to make sense of a profession's ethical relationship with society using a variety of ethical theories. Deontological theories as well as rule-utilitarian viewpoints might account adequately for the ethics of observing the profession's most general promise to society. An ethic of virtue as well as act utilitarianism might also provide a reasonable and illuminating foundation for professional ethics. In the chapters that follow, we make reference to various ethical theories in the attempt to sift through the ethics of professional issues. Fundamentally different opinions about the sources of ethics can nevertheless result in the same conclusion about the ethical course of action. Unfortunately, these different opinions can result in substantial ethical disagreement among members of a profession.

For Further Discussion

1. Consider the following case:

Nurse N, who is employed by a home health agency, is working with a discharge planning team to prepare a young male AIDS victim for discharge from a local community hospital. The patient will be returning to his parents' home. He requests that his parents not be told of his condition, as he has never discussed his homosexuality with them. His home care will require some special techniques in which the family should be instructed.

Analyze this case from each of the ethical perspectives discussed in the present chapter.

2. Chapter 1 argued that profession is a form of commitment or promising. Use each of the sources for ethics discussed in the present chapter as a basis for explaining how this commitment is a matter of *ethical* importance.

Bibliography

Aquinas, T. Edited and annotated by Pegis, A. (1945). Basic Writings of Saint Thomas Aquinas. New York: Random House.

Aristotle. Nichomachean Ethics. Edited and translated by Oswald, M. (1962). Indianapolis: Bobbs-Merrill.

Ashley, B. M. and O'Rourke, K. D. (1978). Health Care Ethics: A Theological Analysis. St. Louis: Catholic Health Association.

Beauchamp, T. L. and Childress, J. F. (1983). Principles of Biomedical Ethics. 2nd edition. New York: Oxford University Press.

Benjamin, M. and Curtis, J. Virtue and the Practice of Nursing. In Shelp, E. (1985). Virtue and Medicine: Explorations in the Character of Medicine. Boston: D. Reidel Publishing Company.

Bentham, J. (1789). An Introduction to the Principles of Morals and Legislation.

Bok, S. (1974). The ethics of giving placebos. Scientific American, 231:17.

Brody, H. (1977). Placebos and the Philosophy of Medicine: Clinical, Conceptual, and Ethical Issues. Chicago: University of Chicago Press.

Dworkin, R. M. (1977). Taking Rights Seriously. Cambridge, Massachusetts: Harvard University Press.

Feinberg, J. (1970). Doing and Deserving. Princeton, New Jersey: Princeton University Press.

Fletcher, J. (1966). Situation Ethics: The New Morality. Philadelphia: Westminster Press.

Frankena, W. K. (1973). Ethics. 2nd edition. Englewood Cliffs, New Jersey: Prentice-Hall, Inc.

Fromm, E. (1947). Man for Himself: An Inquiry into the Psychology of Ethics. Greenwich, Connecticut: Fawcett Publications.

Green, R. M. (1985). Contemporary Jewish Bioethics: A Critical Assessment. In Shelp, Earl E. Theology and Bioethics. Boston: D. Reidel Publishing Company.

Hall, E.W. (1968). The 'Proof' of Utility in Bentham and Mill. Reprinted in Bayles, M., editor. Contemporary Utilitarianism. New York: Doubleday.

Hare, R. M. (1952). The Language of Morals. Oxford, England: Oxford University Press.

Kant, I. Foundations of the Metaphysics of Morals. Edited with an introduction by Beck, L.W. (1959). Indianapolis: Bobbs-Merrill.

MacIntyre, A. C. (1981). After Virtue: A Study in Moral Theory. Notre Dame, Indiana: University of Notre Dame Press.

Mill, J. S. (1863). Utilitarianism. Chicago: H. Regnery Company (1949).

Niebuhr, R. (1935). An Interpretation of Christian Ethics. New York: Harper and Row.

Ozar, D. (1986). Rights: What They Are and Where They Come From. In Werhane, P., Gini, A.R., and Ozar, D., editors (1986). Philosophical Issues in Human Rights. New York: Random House.

Ramsey, P. (1970). The Patient as Person. New Haven: Yale University Press.

Rogers, C. (1961). On Becoming a Person. Boston: Houghton Mifflin Company.
Ross, W. D. (1939). Foundations of Ethics. Oxford, England: Oxford University Press.
Ross, W. D. (1930). The Right and the Good. Oxford, England: Oxford University Press.
Shelp, E. E., editor (1985). Theology and Bioethics. Boston: D. Reidel Publishing Company.
Shelp, E. E., editor (1985). Virtue and Medicine: Explorations in the Character of Medicine. Boston: D. Reidel Publishing Company.
Smart, J. J. C. and Williams, B. (1973). Utilitarianism: For and Against. Cambridge, England: Cambridge University Press.
Steele, S. M. and Harmon, V. M. (1979). Values Clarification in Nursing. New York: Appleton-Century-Crofts.
Veatch, R. (1979). Against Virtue: A Deontological Critique of Virtue Theory in Medical Ethics. In Shelp, E., editor (1979). Virtue and Medicine. Boston: D. Reidel Publishing Company.
Wallace, J. D. (1978). Virtues and Vices. Ithaca, New York: Cornell University Press.

Chapter Three

AUTONOMY AND ETHICS

Autonomy, put simply, is control over one's own life. The word comes from two Greek words that together literally mean "self-rule." An ethical principle of respect for human autonomy deserves our study here for several reasons. First, ethics, from whatever perspective it is viewed, presumes that human beings are capable of self-determination, of acting on principles they adopt as their own. The very possibility of any ethics whatsoever presumes that human beings are autonomous in this way, that they are capable of choosing the principles by which they live. Respect for autonomy is thus a fundamental way of respecting persons as persons.

Second, health care professionals need to take a special interest in the ethical issues surrounding human autonomy. The power that professionals wield and the dependence of the typical patient result in numerous opportunities for violating the autonomy of patients. But the professional also has unique opportunities to *promote* and *protect* human autonomy. This chapter will explore the nature of autonomy, its ethical significance, and the relation of professional nursing to human autonomy.

> This morning when nurse N. met with social worker W. to complete their patient's discharge planning, she sensed something wrong in this case. The patient had originally planned to go home. His plan seemed realistic, given his progress in recovering from a stroke. There was no reason to think that he was incapable of making such a decision or of living with its consequences. But now he states he wants to enter a nursing home. The evening shift staff nurse reported in her notes that yesterday evening during a visit from his two adult children there was a loud discussion. The patient seemed anxious after the family had left but refused her offer to discuss the situation. N. and W. agree that they cannot yet complete the discharge plan.

The nurse and the social worker are reluctant to complete the discharge plan because they suspect that the decision to enter a nursing home might not have been made autonomously. The patient's new decision contradicted what he had previously decided. Certainly a person can change his mind and still be acting autonomously. However, in this case, the events reported by the evening shift nurse made the discharge planners suspect that the patient was being pressured to change his mind. Respect for the patient's autonomy made them reluctant to accept the change of mind as the patient's own decision. But the same respect for autonomy prevented them from assuming that it was *not* the patient's own decision. Not knowing what transpired between the patient and his relatives, they cannot yet draw conclusions. Respect for his autonomy requires that they get more information and a better understanding of the situation. Until they do so, they cannot decide what course of action would most respect the patient.

N. and W. responded on the basis of the ethical principle of respect for human autonomy. Their ethical principle implicitly presumes a certain view of the nature of human beings. Human beings are capable of developing their own goals, desires, and preferences. They can process information in order to arrive at decisions about how to achieve those goals. This process includes both reasoning and choosing. Any time that this process is disrupted there is some question about whether the person is acting autonomously. Persons not acting autonomously are not acting in their fullest human capacities.

A person may fail to act autonomously for any of a number of reasons. Sometimes persons simply do not have the information they need to arrive at a decision. At other times they do not have the ability to process the information. Such a disability is usually called *noncompetence* or *incompetence*. The very young are often presumed to be noncompetent, as are the unconscious and the profoundly retarded. The legal system protects the best interests of a person found to be incompetent by appointing a substitute (a "proxy") to act for the incompetent person in decision making. Persons who are competent in the eyes of the law are not always fully capable of acting autonomously without some assistance. Thus, legal judgments of competence are not always sure guides to respecting a patient's autonomy. In the case under discussion here, the patient's competence is not being questioned. The concern is that some outside pressure (from the family members) may have been so great that the patient was not able to decide as he would have chosen to. Such pressure is called *coercion*.

When N. and W. suspected that their patient's decision was being imposed on him, unquestioning acceptance of his change of mind would have amounted to a lack of concern for his human capabilities, a lack of concern for him as a person. They may well have considered this unethical, no matter what their own ethical orientation, for the principle of respect for human autonomy is not the sole property of only one view of ethics. A utilitarian, for example, might believe that happiness is best obtained by the full use of our powers of autonomous choice (Mill, 1859). A deontological point of view might instead hold that respect for autonomy is a duty that we owe to all other human beings. A theory that emphasizes virtue and human development might hold that the failure to employ all the distinctive capacities with which human beings are gifted amounts to a waste of our human potential.

The ethical principle of respect for human autonomy does not presume that people will always make the best decisions for themselves if they are just left alone. Experience shows that we often fail to decide what is best for ourselves: we fail to buckle our seat belts; we smoke; we overeat; we do all kinds of things that we know and admit to be inconsistent with our own goals in life. This fact gives rise to one disturbing feature about unqualified respect for human autonomy. Respect includes acknowledging the person's freedom to adopt goals with which we disagree, to make decisions that will not lead to the goal adopted or that will have undesired effects.

For a case in point, consider the dilemma of treating a Jehovah's Witness. Members of this religious group refuse blood transfusions because of their interpretation of certain passages in the Old Testament (Dixon and Smalley, 1981). There have been numerous cases of Witnesses who seek treatment but who nevertheless consider themselves morally compelled to reject transfusions that might make surgery possible or even save their lives. Professionals face a dilemma in such cases. To respect the patient's decision to refuse a transfusion restricts the professional's efforts to do everything possible for the patient's recovery. To administer the transfusion against the patient's wishes violates the patient's autonomy.

Sometimes the matter has been turned over to a court of law, with a request that the patient be considered incompetent to make this decision and that a temporary guardian be appointed to make the decision that would be in the patient's best interests. When this strategy is successful, the guardian has the legal power to decide for the patient that he will or will not have the transfusion. Judging another person incompetent should not be taken lightly; the unusualness of a person's value system and ethical principles do not always indicate that the person is not capable of reasoning toward an autonomous decision. When such cases go to court, the decision is not a foregone conclusion. Some courts refuse to intervene; others will do so.

When respect for autonomy conflicts with some other important principle, resolution of the conflict requires some sophistication in our ability to think about ethics. A constructive beginning would be always to deal with autonomy issues as requiring the *burden of proof* to be on those who would choose intervention over respect for autonomy. The concept of burden of proof is fundamental to legal thinking, but it has use in ethical thinking as well. In the criminal law system of the United States, a person is (at least in theory) presumed innocent until proven guilty. This basic presumption determines the process by which the court makes a decision. Accusers must provide evidence to justify their accusation; they are said to "bear the burden of proof."

An analogous presumption is useful in ethics when a person's autonomy conflicts with the attempts of other persons to observe some other important ethical principle. This proposal makes the principle of respect for autonomy paramount in ethics. This is consistent with the role that respect for autonomy occupies in most important ethical theories. It is also consistent with the view that independent decision-making is a fundamental characteristic of human beings.

If the burden of proof is on anyone who would violate another's autonomy in order to favor some other moral principle, autonomy will always at least be considered. But deciding where the burden of proof should lie creates only a *structure* for considering ethical issues. One must still determine what reasons might be sufficiently compelling to override the principle of respect for autonomy. The reasons usually given are themselves competing ethical principles. Although a variety of reasons may be given for violating autonomy, we will discuss two of the ones that recur most often in discussions of health care issues. These are the harm principle and the principle of paternalism.

THE HARM PRINCIPLE

In Chapter 2 we saw that some deontologists (such as Ross) would claim that we have a duty to avoid doing harm to others, a duty of nonmaleficence. Sometimes this duty is interpreted even more broadly as a duty to prevent other persons from harming a third party. Prevention of harm to others is sometimes considered sufficient reason for limiting a person's autonomy. In health care, actions such as involuntary hospitalization of the violent and mentally ill person, required vaccinations, and even denying driver's licenses because of health problems are often justified by an appeal to the harm principle.

One who believes in the harm principle judges that the potential harm that a person may do to others is a serious enough reason to justify an infringement on that person's autonomy. Such judgments cannot be made easily. Judgments about what will happen in the future always involve some uncertainty. In spite of these problems in the use of the harm principle, it still has an important place in our ethical reasoning. In order to achieve any degree of social harmony at all, our society continuously engages in a sort of balancing act, always trying to weigh the right to autonomy against its potential effects on the welfare of others.

THE PRINCIPLE OF PATERNALISM IN HEALTH CARE

The harm that persons can do to themselves is sometimes given as a reason for restricting them. This is different from the harm principle, which would limit one person's autonomy to prevent harm to *others*. Justifying a restriction on autonomy to prevent self-harm is paternalistic. The principle of *paternalism* holds that there are two reasons that would justify restricting another person's autonomy. One is preventing the persons whose autonomy is restricted from doing harm to themselves. The other reason is to ensure some benefit to the person whose autonomy is restricted. A paternalistic action is really a special instance of the more general ethical principles of doing good and preventing harm to others. But it is an application of these principles in a situation in which they conflict with a third very important principle, the principle of respect for autonomy. The issues surrounding paternalism are complex. Because of their complexity and the regularity with which they occur in health care, they deserve our careful analysis.

> Mr. Rice is 80 years old. He came to the hospital with pneumonia. He has severe arthritis, and his eyesight is poor. His daughter reports that he has a history of falls at home, and the family usually assists him in ambulating. The night nurse reports that three times during the night he attempted to use the bathroom unassisted. She suggests that he be restrained. Mary Jones, his primary nurse, must decide whether to request a physician's order for patient restraint.

A restraint that would prevent Mr. Rice from getting out of bed when he chooses would protect him from the harm that he might do to himself. But a restraint would also limit his freedom to move when he chooses. If Nurse Jones requests the restraint, she is judging that protecting Mr. Rice from harm is more important than respecting his right to get out of bed when he wants. What appears at first to be a simple clinical judgment turns out also to be an ethical judgment by the nurse.

In fact, a fall by Mr. Rice would be likely to harm him, but it would probably also affect his family, the staff who care for him, the other patients, the hospital itself, and all those who fund his care. Actions that appear to be paternalistic often are justified by effects other than the benefit of the person whose autonomy is restricted. Here we are concerned with one aspect of the problem: if there were no effects on others, would the welfare of Mr. Rice be a strong enough reason for restraining him? The answer to this question depends on his competence, so we will examine it under several different assumptions.

Suppose Mr. Rice is fully capable of knowing the consequences of not being restrained and of being restrained and is able to communicate his desire not to be restrained. As long as he is capable of understanding and choosing, there is no reason to presume that others can make choices for his welfare better than he can. The principle of paternalism should not be used to override the decisions of persons who are able to know what they want and to make decisions for themselves. In the long run, it *might* be justifiable to request the restraint, but that decision would have to come from some principle other than paternalism.

On the other hand, there is a chance that Mr. Rice is truly incompetent to make decisions for himself. This would be the case if he cannot understand his present situation and the available alternatives or cannot formulate his own preferences and goals. If this is so, someone else will have to make the decision for him. The problem then will be *how* to make the decision.

In trying to make such decisions, persons often resort to a method that resembles the Golden Rule: they consider what they would want done to themselves if they were in the patient's situation. There is some value to this approach; it at least recognizes that the patient is a person, just as the person making the decision is a person. Nurse Jones might try to picture herself in a similar situation and try to determine what *she* would want if she were thinking rationally. She might conclude that a rational person who is interested in preserving his own autonomy would want to be protected from a hip fracture that would ultimately cause a greater loss of autonomy. Still, if Nurse Jones requests restraints on the basis of what she as a rational person would want for herself, she might end up imposing only her own preferences on Mr. Rice. It is notoriously difficult to draw the line between what every rational person would want and what we actually want for ourselves.

The two ways in which we have imagined this case presume that Mr. Rice is either competent or incompetent and that the ethical decisions somehow depend on those categories. In reality, even if persons can be categorized as competent or incompetent, that does not solve the problem of respecting their autonomy. Decisions regarding a person who formerly was competent but has lost that competence can still respect that person's autonomy without assuming that he is now competent. It is often possible to discover what that person would decide for himself if he were now competent. Conversations with family, nonverbal messages, and patient histories all can help reveal a patient's preferences. The Living Will legislation enacted in many states is one example of an institutionalized effort to ensure that the autonomy of persons will be respected even when they become incompetent in the course of a terminal illness. Children, too, may not be capable of making decisions entirely for themselves, but they often are capable of actively participating in decisions that affect them.

Persons always exist with varying capabilities for control over their own lives. The ability to use information to make decisions is acquired only gradually in life and can be lost partially or completely, temporarily or permanently. The ability to have preferences and desires in life is not always gained or lost at the same time as the ability to decide. Both are important to human autonomy. The professional who is sincerely and attentively respectful of human autonomy will respect decisions when the patient can make them but still respect desires and preferences when the patient cannot. Moreover, the recognition that human autonomy is itself good may impel a professional to go beyond respecting autonomy in order to encourage and help develop autonomy.

THE PROFESSIONAL AS A THREAT TO AUTONOMY

Professionals, despite good intentions, may end up restricting patient autonomy more than can be justified ethically. The very nature of the professions makes them a potential threat to autonomy. An occupational group is considered a profession only when its members are widely believed to be experts in an area of human knowledge that other members of society need but cannot readily learn for themselves. This dependence on the expertise of others is an implicit threat to the autonomy of clients or patients. The professions are therefore given a "contract" with society in exchange for their commitment to use their expertise ethically and to the benefit of their clients.

Expertise and Autonomy

The complex and important knowledge that professionals possess can lead them to make unwarranted assumptions about the kinds of expertise that their knowledge gives them. To see this we will examine some issues related to treatment of breast tumors.

At least through the middle of this century it was common for a surgeon to insist on completing both a biopsy and a radical mastectomy on a patient at one time, so that the patient would undergo anesthesia only once. As a result, the patient was often anesthetized for a biopsy and woke up missing a breast. The patient could not use the information gained from the biopsy to make her own decision about what to do next. A patient who might prefer to choose a different surgeon, to refuse surgery, or even to take a few days to prepare herself for a major alteration of her body was not given the opportunity to make a choice. Physicians argued that every additional procedure could itself spread cancer cells, that time was of the essence, and that anesthesia undergone twice was too risky. Assume, for the sake of analysis, that the surgeon's assessment of the risk was well founded. (In fact, although some controversy still remains about what procedures ensure the best prognosis, this particular approach is rarely justified in current practice [Moxley *et al.*, 1980]).

One dangerous assumption by professionals is that their professional knowledge is the only knowledge needed to make decisions for their patients. Health care professionals often understand better than patients do the full clinical implications of health risks, for they have seen the clinical results of risk taking. But the clinical results of a course of action are only a part of its total actual results. A mastectomy can have a variety of effects on the patient and on other people, only some of which are clinical. To a patient, decisions about a clinical procedure are not just clinical decisions; they are decisions that affect the whole person. Professionals may ignore the numerous other factors that individuals consider in making decisions about their lives. When treatment decisions are made without the active participation of the patient, these other relevant areas of knowledge may be lost. Clinical expertise is not expertise about a person's whole life. The assumption that it is can lead to violations of patient autonomy in the name of professional knowledge.

A second assumption, that knowledge of the facts is all one needs to be able to judge the rationality of a risk, is just as threatening to patient autonomy. Knowing what the risks are (both clinical and nonclinical) does not entitle the surgeon to draw conclusions about whether taking the risk would be rational for the patient. To judge the rationality of risk-taking in any context, one needs to know the *importance* of the alternatives and their consequences to the person undergoing the risk. A woman who does not seem to understand the seriousness of refusing to have a mastectomy may have strong feelings about losing her breast. The risk of a possible reduced life span may in fact be less important to her than the feared rejection by loved ones and the loss of sexuality and attractiveness. The same question of importance must arise even if the contemplated procedure is something less radical, for example, a lumpectomy. Clinical expertise does not give the professional knowledge of the importance of such matters. Only patients can give that knowledge. To assume otherwise is to violate their autonomy.

Professional knowledge is essential to professional practice but becomes dangerous when its proper place is misunderstood. Professional knowledge does not substitute for knowledge about the nonclinical areas of a patient's life. Nor does it entitle the professional to draw conclusions about how important some event should be in the patient's life. Failure to realize the limits of professional knowledge leads to violations of the patient's autonomy.

Respect for autonomy is important to ethics in general and to professional ethics in particular, but making it the *only* guiding principle in professional life would lead to a misconstrual of the nature of professional life. The professional would become nothing more than a paid technician who simply does what the patient demands. Professional commitment involves more than the willingness to use expertise as one is told to. It involves also the commitment to use knowledge in the best interests of the patient.

The nurse who deals with a noncompliant patient faces a conflict between two important ethical principles: the principle of respect for autonomy (which would uphold the right of the patient to do as he chooses) and the principle of beneficence (by which the nurse has a duty to serve the best interests of the patient). Patients often are the best judge of what is in their own best interests, but their relationship with a professional also presumes that they can *trust* the professional to act in their best interests. A patient who expects services but makes no use of the professional's knowledge is not entering into a true professional relationship. If efforts to re-establish that relationship fail, then the professional may ultimately be justified in terminating the relationship. The professional's duty certainly requires that she make serious efforts to salvage the relationship, so that she can offer professional care and the patient can still lead an autonomous life. But sometimes ending the relationship may be the only way to respect both the patient's autonomy and the professional's commitment. Chapter 10 presents a more thorough discussion of this issue.

THE PROFESSIONAL AS ADVOCATE FOR AUTONOMY

Persons who seek the services of a professional are already dependent: the professional has some special skill or knowledge that they need and cannot provide for themselves. Other social institutions reinforce this dependence by requiring that certain goods and services be provided only through licensed professionals. Pharmaceuticals, surgery, legal representation, and elementary and secondary education are all restricted in some way so that they are provided only by those with certified skills. The dependence inherent in the professional-client relationship can threaten the autonomy of the patient or client, even when the professional recognizes the ethical importance of respecting human autonomy. The situation of the professions requires an approach to respect for autonomy that goes beyond what might legitimately be expected of private persons in society. The commitment of the professional requires something more than avoiding interference with the autonomy of patients; it requires becoming an *advocate* for them. In this section, we will explore the role of the professional as an advocate for the autonomy of her client.

A person recognized as sick undergoes a transformation both in self-perception and in perception by others. This transformation is important to understand here, because it makes the ill person even more dependent and vulnerable than other persons in society and other users of health services. Parsons has summarized these changes in a description of what he calls the "sick role." In social life, persons often have perceptions and expectations of how others will act or how it would be proper for them to act. Parsons uses the idea of a role to explain the kinds of perceptions and expectations that society has of a person once he is characterized as ill:

> 1. The sick person has not only a right but an obligation to be exempt from normal social role responsibilities.
>
> 2. The sick person is not in control of his own illness. He cannot get well simply by wanting or choosing to.
>
> 3. Sick persons ought to want to get well.
>
> 4. Sick persons have an obligation to seek technically competent help (Parsons and Schutz, 1978).

Sick persons entering a health care system suffer all the disability and loss of autonomy that result from illness. In addition, their autonomy is further limited by the social role they are expected to assume. Well persons who enter the health care system are often expected to assume the same social role, so that they often suffer the same loss of autonomy as an ill person. Wellness programs are often designed to minimize the loss of autonomy to a well person seeking health care assistance. Nevertheless, all who use health care services, whether ill or well, are subjected to a situation in which they seek knowledge and services that they cannot provide for themselves. Leah Curtin has summarized this situation well:

> Whether we as health professionals want it or not, whether we like it or not, we exercise enormous power over those whom we should serve (Curtin, 1979).

The present volume refers to the users of health professional services alternately as "patients" and as "clients." The vacillation in terminology is intentional. The term "patient" has by custom brought with it connotations of the sick role and all the passivity and lack of autonomy associated with it. To refer to users as "clients" invites a comparison of them with those who use the services of other professions. Lawyers, accountants, and architects all have "clients" rather than "patients," and their clients are usually considered autonomous persons seeking expert assistance. Many of the users of health care are more like clients than they are like patients, and the change of terminology may serve as a reminder of this. Still, the fact of illness may result in a person needing the protection (and even the paternalism) that is shown to a patient. Whether one is caring for a patient or a client is a substantive question. Lurking behind the variations in terminology is a serious ethical question related as much to human autonomy as it is to semantics.

Private persons are often able to respect the autonomy of others simply by not becoming involved in their lives. Professionals literally promise to become involved in the lives of their clients. The problem for professional ethics is how to offer services to those who depend on them while still respecting autonomy. The condition of the patient, the structure of the health care system, and the professional relationship itself all make this difficult. Recent philosophical perspectives on nursing have tried to define the appropriate relationship of nursing to human autonomy by appealing to the concept of *advocacy* (Smith, 1980). We will look briefly at two conceptions of the nurse that are antithetical to the claim that the nurse is an advocate. Then we will look more closely at advocacy.

The Handmaiden. The image of the nurse as a servant to the physician has been common throughout this century in the minds of the public, in the expectations of some physicians, and even in the way some nurses think of themselves. Nurses who think of themselves as handmaidens are necessarily prevented from seriously addressing the problem of providing professional service while respecting autonomy. The handmaiden has already acknowledged that it is not her proper place to exercise independent professional judgment or to take independent action on the behalf of her patients. In fact, a handmaiden has no patients; she serves the physician, who serves the patient.

The Surrogate Mother. To claim that nursing is a true profession is to claim that the nurse's primary loyalty is to patients and that her primary duty is to care for patients. Whatever loyalty is owed to the physician is owed only because of the patients. The surrogate mother role proposes a particular way of providing care to patients. In this role the nurse acts in the patients' best interests, but the relationship is similar to the mother-child relationship (Ashley, 1976; Smith, 1980). Such a relationship recognizes both the actual dependence of the patient and the nurse's duty to provide care. But the relationship embodies the female equivalent of paternalism: the nurse decides what is best for the patient just as the mother decides what is best for the child.

The Nurse as Advocate. Neither the handmaiden nor the surrogate mother is capable of fully respecting the autonomy of patients. The idea of advocacy is a basic philosophy of professional patient care. It recognizes the patient's actual dependence and the obligation to respect autonomy while providing care. Instead of "taking care of" patients as the surrogate mother might do or "helping the physician take care of" them as the handmaiden might do, the nurse as advocate *cares for* patients. The idea of "caring for" has been aptly described by Milton Mayeroff:

> To care for another person, in the most significant sense, is to help him grow and actualize himself (Mayeroff, 1971, p. 1).

To accomplish this, Mayeroff says, we must

> . . . be able to be *with* him in his world, "going" into his world in order to sense from "inside" what life is like for him, what he is striving to be, and what he requires to grow (p. 42).

Caring for another requires recognizing what the other is striving for, the goals and values that the other considers important. The advocate takes the part of the person served and uses her professional expertise to aid him in growing. What the patient is striving to be determines what counts as progress or growth for the patient. Caring always involves respect for the person's own chosen direction.

Certainly, all professionals should be advocates; to say this is to say only that they should respect the autonomy of their clients while in their professional roles. All the professions must determine precisely how their particular professional service can be combined with advocacy. The definition of nursing proposed in the Social Policy Statement (see Chapter 1) implies that the role of nursing is to ensure that the patient is able to integrate his health status with a continued autonomous life.

Nurses frequently lack authority in the health hierarchy. This can be both an impediment and an aid to their efforts to be advocates. Nurses do not always have the authority to deal with their patients as they would choose to. But at the same time, nurses are often seen as less authoritarian than are physicians. This perception, coupled with the intimate contact that nurses have with hospitalized patients, can put the nurse in a unique position to know the patient, his goals, hopes, and fears. The nurse is often able to enter into the world of the patient, as Mayeroff urges, to engage the patient in a dialogue between equals. The nurse can learn from this encounter what an autonomous life means to this particular patient and can join this understanding to knowledge of how the patient's illness can threaten this autonomy. Nurses who know how to listen to patients and how to understand what they hear and who are prepared to initiate action as a result can serve as advocates in a unique and powerful way.

Enhancing a patient's autonomy requires not withholding information, but it also requires providing information in a way that enables the patient to use it. Thus patient education is more than an item in a job description, more than a task that nurses take on because no one else is doing it. It is an attempt to respect the patient's autonomy while honoring the fundamental commitment of the nurse to advocacy.

In a society where persons who seek health care are relegated to the sick role, a person who supports the autonomy of the ill is likely to meet with resistance. If there is a customary perception of the appropriate role of the sick, there is a corresponding customary role for those who care for the sick. True efforts to serve as an advocate must go beyond the clinical interactions of the nurse and take a broader view, a view of professional issues. It is naive, simplistic, and false to believe that a person can be an ethical nurse with her eyes focused on nothing beyond the clinical procedure she is performing.

The issues are complex: they are compounded out of problems internal to the nursing profession as well as problems in the larger society and other social institutions. In facing these problems, it is easy to diagnose oneself as powerless and to retreat into what Rollo May has called "pseudoinnocence":

> When we face questions too big and too horrendous to contemplate . . . we tend to shrink into this kind of innocence and make a virtue of powerlessness, weakness, and helplessness . . . . With unconscious purpose we close our eyes to reality and persuade ourselves that we have escaped it (May, 1972, pp. 49-50).

But such pseudoinnocence cuts a person off from the real world, the one in which we all live and act and make our plans and commitments. The ability to make a commitment is the exercise of a marvelous human capacity, and to make a commitment to the service of human life is to celebrate life itself.

For Further Discussion

1. Return to the brief case of restraints for Mr. Rice as described in this chapter. What other kinds of effects on other people should Nurse Jones consider in deciding whether to request restraints for him? What kinds of effects do you think are important enough to justify restraining him against his will?

2. Living Will legislation was mentioned in this chapter as a way of respecting the autonomy of persons who were competent but are no longer. Explain how this is so. Does your state have a Living Will provision? How would Living Will legislation affect nursing practice in the care of the terminally ill patient? Are there any dangers that Living Will legislation would result in restricting a person's autonomy?

3. Use the discussion of ethics, expert knowledge, and advocacy to develop an ethical position on the nursing care of a Jehovah's Witness refusing a needed transfusion.

Bibliography

Ashley, J. A. (1976). Hospitals, Paternalism and the Role of the Nurse. New York: Teachers' College Press.

Brodegard, N. F. (1982). The Nurse Defined as Symbiotic Mother. In Muff, J., Editor (1982). Socialization, Sexism and Stereotyping: Women's Issues in Nursing. St. Louis: C.V. Mosby Company.

Childress, J. F. (1982). Who Should Decide? Paternalism in Health Care. New York: Oxford Univerity Press.

Cross, A. W. and Churchill, L. R. (1982). Ethical and Cultural Dimensions of Informed Consent. Annals of Internal Medicine, 96: 110-113.

Curtin, L. (1979). The Nurse as Advocate: A Philosophical Foundation for Nursing. Advances in Nursing Science, 1:1. p. 6.

Davis, A. J. and Aroskar, M. A. (1983). Ethical Dilemmas and Nursing Practice, 2nd Edition. Norwalk, Connecticut: Appleton-Century-Crofts.

Dixon, J. L. and Smalley, M. G. (1981). Jehovah's Witnesses. JAMA, 246(21): 2471-2472, November 27.

Gadow, S. (1980). Existential Advocacy: Philosophical Foundation of Nursing. In Spicker, S. and Gadow, S., Editors (1980). Nursing: Images and Ideals. New York: Springer.

Gert, B. and Culver, C. M. (1976). Paternalistic Behavior. Philosophy and Public Affairs, 6: 45-57.

Ingelfinger, F. (August 31, 1972). Informed (But Uneducated) Consent. New England Journal of Medicine, 287: 455-456.
Kohnke, M. F. (1982). Advocacy: Risk and Reality. St. Louis: C.V. Mosby Company.
May, R. (1972). Power and Innocence: A Search for the Sources of Violence. New York: W.W. Norton, pp. 49-50.
Mayeroff, M. (1971). On Caring. New York: Harper and Row, p. 1; p. 42.
Mill, J. S. (1859). On Liberty. New York: Liberal Arts Press, 1956.
Moxley, J. H., Allegro, J. C., Henney, J., and Muggia, F. M. (1980). Treatment of Primary Breast Cancer. JAMA, 244: 797-800.
Parsons, T. and Schutz, A. (1978). Theory of Social Action. Bloomington: Indiana University Press.
Ramsey, P. (1970). The Patient as Person. New Haven: Yale University Press.
Sartorius, R. (editor) (1984). Paternalism. Minneapolis: University of Minnesota Press.
Smith, S. (1980). Three Models of the Nurse-Patient Relationship. In Spicker, S. and Gadow, S., editors (1980). Nursing: Images and Ideals. New York: Springer.

Chapter Four

PROFESSIONAL ISSUES IN CLINICAL ETHICS

Although professional issues are often regarded as something apart from both ethical issues and clinical issues, our announced agenda in this book is to show that this separation is artificial. Clinical issues, professional issues, and ethical issues are so thoroughly intertwined that it is impossible to think of them and deal with them separately. Ethical problems in clinical practice cannot be solved through the mechanical application of some preferred ethical principle in order to choose the best course of action. Such problems are compounded by the professional-client relationship and by the social environment within which the members of the profession care for patients.

The present chapter examines a case in which clinical and professional issues together create the nurse's actual ethical problem. A case similar to this one was originally reported elsewhere (Carroll and Humphrey, 1979). The insights of ethical theory as well as the understanding of professional commitment will clarify the situation.

Although this chapter proceeds in a way intended to help the nurse *understand* the various dimensions of the ethical problem that she faces, it does not offer a mechanical step by step protocol for making ethical decisions. Although such protocols appear to make being ethical somewhat simpler, ethical and professional problems themselves do not always have a single obviously correct solution. In the end, the ethical person must be prepared to live with a certain amount of ambiguity and uncertainty; that subject will be discussed at the end of this chapter.

AN AMBIGUOUS MEDICATION ORDER

Mrs. Brumley was admitted to the hospital two days after her 78th birthday with a diagnosis of metastatic lung cancer. Her general condition had deteriorated rapidly in recent months and Dr. Levy, her physician, expected her to die within a few weeks. Mrs. Brumley was experiencing considerable pain and was requiring more care at home than her daughter was able to provide. Dr. Levy admitted her to try to control the pain more effectively and to give the daughter a much-needed rest. On admission, Dr. Levy ordered Demerol 75 mg every two hours.

Although this was a relatively large dose of Demerol for Mrs. Brumley's size, she tolerated the medication well for the first 24 hours and reported relief of her pain. On the second morning of her hospitalization, when Nurse Munson went to administer the medication, Mrs. Brumley wakened slowly and seemed slightly confused about her surroundings. Her blood pressure had dropped significantly from the day before and her breathing was shallow. She still complained of pain.

Nurse Munson decided not to administer the medication. Instead, she phoned Dr. Levy, reporting the patient's condition and expressing her belief that continuing the medication could be fatal to the patient. Dr. Levy responded with sarcasm that Mrs. Brumley "had such a great life to look forward to." Nevertheless, he changed the Demerol order to PRN.

Meanwhile, Mrs. Brumley continued to complain of pain and requested that the nurse give her the "medicine that was working so well" at controlling her discomfort.

CLINICAL ETHICAL ISSUES

A PRN order has suddenly given Nurse Munson more responsibility than she may have anticipated. A PRN order (*pro re nata* means "as the matter arises") is often used to give the nurse some discretion to alter a physician's order, if the patient's condition should change. When thus used, the PRN order acknowledges the nurse's direct and ongoing knowledge of the patient and her skill in realizing when important changes occur and knowing how to adjust the order accordingly. Used judiciously, the PRN order can work for the benefit of the patient by permitting decisions to be made readily and with up-to-date information. It can also serve to shift the burden of decision-making in a clinically or ethically complex or ambiguous case.

The most pressing reality is that now Nurse Munson must respond somehow to Mrs. Brumley's request for medication. Examination of the courses of action open to her will lead to discussion of several ethical principles that seem consistent with professional ethics and even more fundamental foundations in ethics. The principles of respect for human autonomy and of nonmaleficence will be examined. Issues of utility will arise naturally from that discussion. The simple application of one or another of these principles in the hope of finding the right course of action is too narrow for the situation in which Nurse Munson finds herself. The discussion will be expanded to include other considerations that place this situation in a broader decision-making context.

Initially, Nurse Munson's alternatives appear to be clear-cut: either she can respect Mrs. Brumley's wishes and give her the medication when she requests it or she can refuse Mrs. Brumley's requests and use her own best judgment about the appropriate times and amounts of medication. The physician's PRN order appears to have authorized her to do either of these, using her own professional judgment.

Assume (for the sake of discussion) that respect for the autonomy of the patient should be the sole relevant ethical principle in this case. We have seen that this principle can be both a fundamental way of respecting persons and the object of a special professional commitment by the nurse. How would the principle of autonomy be applied here? It might seem to indicate that Mrs. Brumley should be given the medication when she demands it. That conclusion would assume that Mrs. Brumley's demands truly express her autonomously made choice. To act autonomously, a person must have all the relevant information about alternatives and consequences, be able to clearly formulate personal goals, and be capable of using information and goals to make decisions that will achieve those goals.

There are several reasons for suspecting that Mrs. Brumley's call for medication is not an informed decision by a person acting autonomously and that giving the medication as she requests it would not respect her autonomy. First, it is not obvious that a large dose of Demerol is what she wants. Certainly, she has requested that medication. But her communication with the nurse indicates that what she really seeks is pain relief. She may be operating on an uninformed assumption that the previously prescribed dosage of Demerol is the "right" medicine for her, and that its effectiveness yesterday proves its effectiveness and safety today.

Even if she has accurate information concerning the nature and effects of this medication and of alternative measures, Mrs. Brumley's request for Demerol might still not be an autonomous choice. Her present physical condition (semi-alert, low blood pressure) and the effects of previous medication may leave her able to verbalize a wish but not able to weigh rationally for herself all the information she would normally use in deciding.

Certainly, there is ample reason to suspect that Mrs. Brumley's initial request for Demerol should not be taken immediately and uncritically as an informed choice by a fully autonomous person. A nurse who considers it her duty to be an advocate for the patient's autonomy would find in this an indication of what her next course of action should be. The nurse would have to spend adequate time with Mrs. Brumley to develop a judgment about her cognitive status. If she is competent to make a judgment, the nurse would still have to educate her to ensure that she has relevant information and understands it well enough to use it in making a choice. This would be the ideal function of *advocacy* in such a case.

However, time spent with Mrs. Brumley is time not spent with some other patient. In choosing to spend additional nursing time advocating for Mrs. Brumley, Nurse Munson will be choosing how best to use a scarce resource. On a very personal level, she is involved in a decision about how to allocate a limited amount of available health care. She may choose to respond to this problem of how to ration her time by asking the kind of question that the utilitarian sees at the heart of ethics: which course of action will yield the best consequences? To answer such a question, she would have to know the alternative uses of her nursing time (the other patients, their conditions, and possible nursing interventions) and the relative value of those outcomes.

Policies and procedures within the hospital may limit and channel the nurse's problem of time allocation. Staffing policies, for example, will determine the total number of nurses assigned to the unit on the basis of the number of patients and the severity of their conditions. Such policies ordinarily assume a certain average number of nursing care hours per patient, but they do not dictate the actual amount of time to be spent with each patient. Other policies and procedures specify the minimum care to be given to each patient. They may specify how often a nurse must see each patient, how often an IV site should be changed, and related matters. All such policies limit the individual nurse's freedom to allocate care as she chooses.

The existence of relevant policies will not solve Nurse Munson's problem here. Instead, it shows that her ethical and professional judgment about how best to allocate nursing resources cannot be directly acted upon. In order to exercise her professional judgment she must engage in activities designed to influence policies and procedures. These activities may have to be collective; it is unlikely that a hospital staff nurse will change policies and procedures without the cooperation of others. It is also unlikely that she will be aware of all the relevant information that is used in the development of policies and procedures.

Although the problem in this case first appeared to be how best to be an advocate for Mrs. Brumley's autonomy, we see now that the case is more complex than that. Nurse Munson may fully intend to respect autonomy in her professional role as a nurse. Being an advocate involves more than intellectual allegiance to the principle of respect for autonomy when choices must be made. Preserving autonomy requires an allocation of resources. When resources are limited, the nurse makes a decision concerning priorities. When she does so, she works within the confines of established policies and procedures.

Although respect for autonomy and the concern for maximizing utility are both important in this situation, they are not the *only* relevant moral principles. An extremely large dose of pain relief medication to a patient who is already experiencing depressed respiration and changes in blood pressure creates the additional risk of accidentally inducing the death of the patient. Even when the dosage is not great enough to cause death, there is still a danger of inducing drug dependency in the patient. The nurse's reluctance to cause death or addiction may stem from her belief that it is ethically wrong to do harm to other persons. When such a concern is elevated to the level of a moral principle, it is called the principle of *nonmaleficence*.

This principle is supported by a number of ethical theories. Many views of professional ethics, for example, see the professional's duty as above all to do no harm, as stated in the Hippocratic oath. It is reasonable to presume as well that a person following a golden rule ethic would not voluntarily do harm to another. A person who lives by ethical duties (a "deontologist," in the terminology adopted here) is likely to see avoidance of harm to others as one of those duties.

Before discussing how the principle of nonmaleficence applies to this situation, it is important to bring up its counterpart, the principle of *beneficence*, which holds that we ought to do good for others in addition to avoiding harm to them. Not all ethical theories would hold that we have a duty to beneficence; some people believe that in fact our duties to others do not include doing good for them as long as we avoid harming them. However, a person who believes that there is an ethical duty to do good to others would also believe that it would be wrong to do harm to another. However, for the professional, there can be little doubt that there is a duty to do good. Beneficence is, in fact, crucial to the commitment to others that the professional makes.

Although the principles of nonmaleficence and beneficence appear to be clear, when we actually apply them to situations we begin to see problems that were not immediately obvious. First, both of these principles presume some criterion for determining what is good and what is harmful. Even if we could agree on such criteria, these two principles might still conflict with other moral principles we value. In the present situation, efforts to do good and to avoid doing harm may conflict with efforts to respect the patient's autonomy. What Mrs. Brumley would choose for herself is not necessarily what would do her the most good and is possibly something that might cause her harm.

Mrs. Brumley's terminal illness further complicates the problems of determining what would constitute benefit or harm to her. Ordinarily, these principles are applied by mentally judging as "more important" or "less important" the kind of harm that might be caused or the kinds of benefits that might be created by the contemplated course of action. Then the probability that these harms or benefits will occur is considered. It is only at that point that a person can decide what course of action would be most nonmaleficent or most beneficent to the person affected. Although we might ordinarily judge the dangers of drug-induced death or addiction to be so great that the nonmaleficent person would avoid them, Mrs. Brumley's terminal condition may require giving a different weight to them. She is already expected to die in the near future, so the possibility of addiction or drug-induced death may not be the harm to her that they would be to a person with a greater life expectancy. In that case, the benefit of pain relief may outweigh the dangers that it poses.

Whether Nurse Munson could choose a course of medication that places Mrs. Brumley at greater risk is somewhat dependent on the nature of the institution in which she provides care. In a medical-surgical unit of an acute care hospital it may be inappropriate to provide a course of care that shortens the patient's survival while providing immediate comfort. If that is so, then the beneficent nurse will seek to place the patient in a setting more prepared to provide care appropriate to the needs of the terminally ill.

Hospice care is a growing effort to meet the health care needs unique to the terminally ill, but there are difficulties in referring a patient for hospice care. It is not available in every community; insurance coverage for hospice care is inadequate; and entry into a hospice program ordinarily requires an explicit terminal diagnosis and a referral from the attending physician. These are all social policy issues that demand the attention of those who have a professional duty to do good to the terminally ill.

REACHING CONCLUSIONS

We have attempted to survey this case from the standpoint of various ethical principles. We saw that mere accession to Mrs. Brumley's wishes is not the same as respecting her autonomy. We saw also that functioning as an advocate, as demanded by professional ethics, is not itself a clear-cut course of action, and that even if it were, it might conflict with other duties that the nurse has to other patients. We attempted then to look at a duty that is at the basis of utilitarian ethics, beneficence—or the duty to do good to others—and saw again that it was not certain how it should be applied here. Similar problems arose in taking as the guiding principle the duty to nonmaleficence, avoiding harm to others.

We have arrived here at no conclusion about the ethical course of action. That was not the purpose of this case analysis. This case analysis is intended to present some of the issues that professionals face in arriving at ethical decisions and to show some of the impediments to decision-making. As we claimed in earlier chapters, the selection of personal ethical principles is a function of a broader philosophy of life, a view of the nature and purpose of human existence.

Even assuming that we already have a well-considered philosophy of life and know what kind of ethics we thereby become committed to, problems still arise. Professional decisions are not always made individually; they are bound up with attitudes toward nursing, with policies and procedures, and with the availability of alternative resources. Clinical situations and the ethical issues that arise in them are not separable from issues that the profession itself faces.

Nurse Munson might be able to escape this thorny web of issues by passing the problem to another nurse. She could simply refuse to give the medication or could request that someone else be assigned to care for Mrs. Brumley. If she were to do so, she would not have *resolved* the problem but would be attempting to *absolve* herself from it. In effect, she would turn the patient into a "hot potato"—a burning situation best dealt with by passing it on.

The most important result of initiating such a game is that the patient is treated simply as an object rather than as a client to be served by a professional. As a matter of ordinary ethics, we are obligated to treat persons as persons and not as objects only. If the physician's PRN order was really an effort to escape a difficult situation, the professional nurse, as an advocate, has an obligation not only to refuse to play such a game, but to end it for the sake of the patient. When avoiding complexity in a nurse's own life becomes more important than a patient's or client's well-being, the nurse has forgotten what it is to become a member of a profession.

Uncertainty and complexity in decision-making in professional life cannot be avoided. The ethical professional must face them head on. The concluding sections of this chapter explore the fact that there are limits to what we can know and do and how these relate to an ethical professional life.

LIVING WITH UNCERTAINTY

Precise and certain knowledge offers us a certain amount of security. It enables us to direct our own course, to effectively translate our intentions to action. However, when thoughts and actions become shrouded in ambiguity, we feel a loss of control over our own selves; this becomes an important impetus to a search for further knowledge. So there is some positive value even in our uncertainty.

Uncertainty occurs both in knowledge about clinical matters and in ethical thinking. Nurses sometimes must choose from among alternative clinical measures. Although there are often some established criteria for choosing some specific clinical measure, there may sometimes be more than one appropriate measure or the present situation may not exactly match the textbook case. Similarly, clinical uncertainty could arise because of the necessity of acting without complete knowledge.

Ethical decision-making in clinical practice sometimes must proceed under uncertainty that arises from a lack of knowledge of the facts of a situation or from the uniqueness of the situation. In the case discussed in this chapter, for example, Nurse Munson may have needed some specific additional information concerning Mrs. Brumley's real intentions, the likely effect of continuing the medication, the effect that additional time spent with Mrs. Brumley would have on other patients, relevant hospital policies, and the support of the physician and the nurse manager for whatever course of action Nurse Munson chose. In actual life all the desirable information is not always available at the time it is needed, and decisions must be made with the information that is at hand.

In addition to the uncertainty caused by lack of information, the effort to be ethical creates new sources of uncertainty of a different sort. Beginning with the most basic principles or values on which we base our ethics, there is uncertainty. One's selection of ethical principles to live by cannot be proved in the way that the solution to an algebra problem can be proved, so we cannot have the same degree of confidence that we shall be shown to be correct. Principles are closely bound up with fundamental beliefs about the nature of being human, the nature of the world, and the possible ultimate meaning of these. Some of these beliefs and the ethical principles developed from them may be more *reasonable* than others, but their correctness will never be established with absolute certainty either by observation or by deductive proof. We are left, therefore, with an uncertainty at the very heart of life and must choose from among plausible or reasonable philosophies or develop a philosophy based on faith. The ethical principles that we develop from our philosophy are no more certain than the philosophy on which they are based, and these principles raise additional uncertainties about how to apply them to specific situations.

Uncertainty cannot be completely escaped, so one must develop a "philosophy of dealing with uncertainty" in professional practice. The heart of the issue is really in one's attitude toward uncertainty. The professional who accepts uncertainty in practice situations avoids the paralysis that comes from postponing action until all information is available. At the same time, this acceptance involves a danger: it can lead to indifference to new and developing knowledge. For the practicing nurse the result might be falling behind in new clinical skills, refusing to deal with problems of effective communications among health professions, or refusal to sort out difficult but solvable ethical problems.

Those who refuse to deal with ethical problems often support their inaction with the claim that "we all have our own values, and no ethical thinking is any better than any other." Such a view sees only part of the picture. It recognizes that ethics is in one way a personal matter and that there are continuing uncertainties. But it fails to see that ethics is about not only the person who has the values but also about what others are entitled to. A professional simply cannot see ethical values as nothing more than an expression of self; they are also an expression of what is owed to clients. To fail to recognize this ignores the interpersonal aspect of professional commitment and of professional life itself.

Dialogue is an important remedy to uncertainty in ethics. Most of us tend to avoid it, probably because it is considered bad taste to openly air our disagreements about values. But ethical dialogue need not consist of criticizing the people with whom we discuss the problem. It can and should be focused on the problem itself, and especially on the rights of patients in problematic health care situations. Many hospitals are now developing ethics committees and adopting practices such as ethical rounds. The new perspectives that such opportunities for dialogue can create should not be ignored.

Although some value exists in learning to tolerate uncertainty, there is a point at which excessive tolerance amounts to neglect of professional and ethical commitments: to tolerate uncertainty at all times and under all circumstances is to ignore the value of knowledge. There must be a delicate balance between accepting the limits of the human mind's potential for certain knowledge and maintaining the keen edge in ethical thinking and perception that professionals owe to patients. That balance itself is a problem for the ethical profession; it is somewhat uncertain and cannot be embodied in a precise formula. It is wise to remember the advice and example of Aristotle, one of the earliest writers about ethics. He began his discussion of ethics with an admonition:

> Therefore, in a discussion of such subjects . . . we must be satisfied to indicate the truth with a rough and general sketch . . . . For a well-schooled man is one who searches for that degree of precision in each kind of study which the nature of the subject at hand permits . . . (*Nichomachean Ethics*, 1094b, pp. 13-24).

Such advice could serve to excuse one's intellectual laziness. For Aristotle, instead, it invited him to inquire how much precision the subject of ethics *does* permit. In doing so, he wrote a still valuable little book about ethics, the one from which this passage is quoted. Aristotle's example embodies a useful rule of thumb in dealing with uncertainty: we need to be aware of the limits of knowledge, but we must go all the way to the limits rather than making a half-hearted effort to be fully informed.

A second rule of thumb can be helpful in a situation in which one has truly reached the limits of what can be known (either about the facts of the situation or about what ethical principle should be applied). In such situations each possible decision might result in an outcome that one would not choose with perfect and certain knowledge. In such cases a useful principle is that one must determine whether there are outcomes that should *always* be sought or *always* avoided, even if the successful outcome of our actions is uncertain or if other undesirable outcomes might follow. Nurse Munson is in such a situation here: she must determine whether it is so important to respect Mrs. Brumley's request that she should risk the possibility of overmedication. Such a judgment would involve deciding the priority that some principles or values should have over others in our ethics. This second rule assumes that we have clear beliefs about ethics and how to apply ethics to the present situation, and that the only uncertainty is about the empirical outcome of our course of action.

These two rules may sometimes help in making a decision when faced with an uncertainty that cannot be dispelled; at other times they might not. Using such principles does ensure that we will have done the best we can with a situation. There may be times when one must still be left with a residue of uncertainty. We can offer no antidote for that; we can only acknowledge that it does happen. Professionals sometimes assume that the burden of uncertainty is entirely theirs to bear, but in fact the uncertainty relates to the patient's own life. In many cases, the fact that there is uncertainty is a piece of information that the patient needs in order to maintain autonomy.

LIVING WITH UNAVOIDABLE CONSEQUENCES

"I'm caught between a rock and a hard place."

"I'm damned if I do, damned if I don't."

There are other (more colorful) ways of expressing an unpleasant fact that we all must sometimes face. Even the most ethical course of action can have undesirable but unavoidable consequences even when ambiguity and uncertainty do not complicate the problem. Respect for a patient's autonomy can result in decisions on his part that will irreversibly damage his health. Challenging an authority for the sake of the patient can bring repercussions down on the challenger. The list could go on, even with the few cases examined in this volume.

Adverse consequences are not a fate unique to the nurse; anyone who makes decisions and who values some results more than others will sometimes be unavoidably disappointed by results. Intellectually, we all understand that the world cannot be totally remolded to suit the values and principles that we believe should have paramount importance. But to be reminded of this when attempting to make the world a better place is very disconcerting.

Nothing can be done about unavoidable consequences. However, one can pay careful attention to which consequences are labeled as "unavoidable." Most often we think of something avoidable as something that we can personally and individually control. In fact, ethics has by and large been construed as a decision-making process for those situations over which the individual can have some control.

There is another group of consequences that should be considered avoidable. Possible courses of action and their results are shaped not just by the intentions and decisions of the individual actors but by a web of other things, including perceptions and images, customs, legal structures, organizational frameworks, and policies and procedures. These too can change, although the possible changes may involve time and sacrifice on the parts of many persons acting individually and collectively. The problem that Nurse Munson faced in this chapter is compounded by aspects of the situation that she cannot control individually but which can be affected by collective activities. Hospital policies related to allotment of nursing time, the availability of alternative forms of care for the dying, and the legal legitimacy of the PRN order all help to determine what consequences any course of action will have.

Critically examining our conceptions of what is unavoidable is an essential part of an ethical life. Otherwise, ethics is based on a form of self-deceit, a pseudoinnocence that permits escape from action because "there's nothing I can do." Improved personal knowledge and skill and personal and collective activities can alter what would otherwise be unavoidable consequences. Societal institutions seem at first to be uncontrollable. They therefore appear to make personal actions have results that are unintended. Intellectual and ethical honesty require examination of the control that can be exerted over institutional and social conditions that affect professional practice. Honesty requires willingness to make a transition from asking only what "I" can avoid or do to asking what "we" can avoid or do.

It may be disconcerting for a nurse to be argued into broader and broader issues that affect the profession collectively (problems *of nursing* that are not just problems *of nurses*). Those who enter nursing most often expect to help patients on an individual basis. However, as the case examined here shows, to separate the collective professional issues of nursing from the ones that the individual nurse faces is artificial and futile. The day-to-day practice of nursing is dependent upon what nursing is in the employing institution, in the community, in the state, and even in broader society. Nursing can be practiced ethically and professionally in clinical situations only when nurses deal with all the conditions that affect nursing practice.

It would be unrealistic to conclude this chapter without acknowledging that some bad consequences are truly unavoidable despite the best efforts of the skillful individual nurse and the collective efforts of the profession. There is little else that can be said about this fact. But living with truly unavoidable and undesirable consequences is not unique to nursing, to health care, or even to the professions in general. It is the human condition.

Choosing to enter a profession amounts to voluntarily biting off a larger chunk of the human condition. The professional chooses to become involved (with expertise and commitment) in an area of human life in which important elements of human welfare are at stake and in which most people must depend on experts. In making that choice, the professional becomes committed to living with and wrestling with the problem of professional issues and, sometimes, unavoidable consequences.

For Further Discussion

1. Research the philosophy behind the hospice movement. Find out about its policies for pain medication for the dying. Would hospice have been a practical and ethical alternative for Mrs. Brumley? Explain. What current issues related to hospice care are occurring now? How will they affect the nurse's ability to care for patients?

2. Review the two proposed rules of thumb for dealing with uncertainty. Discuss how they might be used in some situation with which you are familiar. Are there other rules you would propose for such situations?

3. At the conclusion of this chapter it was suggested that the development of personal qualities was as important a part of professional ethics as are appropriate principles for decision-making. Such personal qualities for professional life can be called "professional virtues." What personal qualities do you think would be important for a nurse to be able to practice professionally in the kind of situation discussed in this chapter? Why? In preparing your responses, be sure to consider the problems of dealing with uncertainty.

Bibliography

Aroskar, M. (1980). Anatomy of an Ethical Dilemma: The Practice. American Journal of Nursing, 80(4): 661-663, April.

Aroskar, M. (1980). Anatomy of an Ethical Dilemma: The Theory. American Journal of Nursing, 80(4): 658-660, April.

Bandman, E. L. and Bandman, B. (editors) (1978). Bioethics and Human Rights: A Reader for Health Professionals. Boston: Little, Brown and Company.

Benjamin, M. and Curtis, J. (1981). Ethics in Nursing. New York: Oxford University Press.

Caplan, A. L. (1983). Can Applied Ethics Be Effective in Health Care and Should It Strive to Be? Ethics, 93: 311-319, January.

Carroll, M. A. and Humphrey, R. A. (editors) (1979). Moral Problems in Nursing: Case Studies. Washington, D. C.: University Press of America.

Cranford, R. E. and Doudera, A. E. (1984). Institutional Ethics Committees and Health Care Decision Making. Ann Arbor, Michigan: Health Administration Press.

Flaherty, M. J. (1980). Ethical Decision Making in an Interdisciplinary Setting. In Ethics in Nursing Practice and Education. Kansas City, Missouri: American Nurses' Association.

Fromer, M. J. (1980). Teaching Ethics by Case Analysis. Nursing Outlook, 28: 604-609, October.

Henry, C. (1983). The Ethics of Ethics: Nurses' Participation on Ethical Committees. Nursing Mirror, 156(24): 30, June 15.

Holmes, C. (1979). Bioethical Decision-Making: An Approach to Improve the Process. Medical Care, 17(11): 1131-1138, November.

Jameton, A. (1984). Nursing Practice: The Ethical Issues. Englewood Cliffs, New Jersey: Prentice-Hall.

Jonsen, A. R., Siegler, M., and Winslade, W. J. (1982). Clinical Ethics: A Practical Approach to Ethical Decisions in Clinical Medicine. New York: Macmillan Company.

Kestenbaum, V. (editor) (1982). The Humanity of the Ill. Knoxville, Tennessee: University of Tennessee Press.

Lumpp, F. (1979). The Role of the Nurse in the Bioethical Decision-Making Process. Philadelphia: W.B. Saunders Company.

Mazonson, P. D., et al. (1979). Medical Ethical Rounds: Development and Organization. Rocky Mountain Medical Journal, 76(6): 282-288, November-December.

Muyskens, J. L. (1982). Moral Problems in Nursing: A Philosophical Investigation. Totowa, New Jersey: Rowman and Littlefield.

Pinkus, R. L. (1981). Medical Foundations of Various Approaches to Medical-Ethical Decision Making. Journal of Medical Philosophy, 6(3): 295-307, August.

President's Commission for the Study of Ethical Problems in Medicine and Biomedical and Behavioral Research (1982). Making Health Care Decisions. Washington, D.C.: U.S. Government Printing Office.

Robertson, J. A. (1983). The Rights of the Critically Ill. Cambridge, Massachusetts: Ballinger Publishing Company.

Siegler, M. (1982). Decision-Making Strategy for Clinical-Ethical Problems in Medicine. Archives of Internal Medicine, 142(12): 2178-2179, November.

Veatch, R. M. (1977). Case Studies in Medical Ethics. Cambridge, Massachusetts: Harvard University Press.

Weir, R. F. (editor) (1977). Ethical Issues in Death and Dying. New York: Columbia University Press.

Whitman, H. (1980). Ethical Issues in Cancer Nursing. I: Defining the Issues. Oncology Nursing Forum, 7: 37-40, Fall.

Chapter Five

CHOOSING A NURSING ROLE

Roles and jobs are not the same thing. The term "role" is used to describe a way of acting that is appropriate to the relationships that exist in some given social situation (Emmet, 1975). Jobs, on the other hand, focus narrowly on the employer-employee relationship. Most nurses who practice do in fact work for an employer, but that relationship by itself does not adequately portray the complexities of nursing practice. Although most of the practice options discussed in this chapter are in fact choices of jobs, they are approached here as choices of roles as well. In order to know the potential for a truly professional practice, one must examine the web of relationships with which each practice option is involved.

Choosing a role within nursing is partially a matter of taste. Nurses, just as other people, will choose a job within which they can experience satisfaction with their own work. Work is more than a necessity for most human beings; it is a potential source of personal satisfaction, a way of expressing oneself, of becoming part of the world in which one lives.

But when one has already made a nursing commitment, choosing a role also involves value questions related to the professional commitment. The professional nurse faces the problem of remaining true to that commitment to serve patients with expertise, while at the same time experiencing the job satisfaction that human beings legitimately expect for themselves. Little of a general nature can be said about nursing roles and personal satisfaction, for individual preferences vary. However, much can be said about how existing professional roles are related to the ability to fulfill one's commitment. The diversity of contemporary nursing roles creates exciting possibilities for the new graduate as well as for the experienced nurse making a job change. It also presents a confusing array of choices and questions for the nurse to reflect upon in deciding how and where she will practice her profession.

Several different forces have made the choice of a nursing role more complex than ever before. First, the practice opportunities that now exist require kinds and levels of skill uncommon several decades ago. Technological changes in health care and increased emphasis on wellness have contributed to the development of new areas of specialization, each involving particular skills and knowledge. Recent efforts at cost containment have created a demand for assurance that quality will be retained, and nurses often function in positions related to quality assurance and utilization review.

Second, the job-seeking nurse has become progressively more career-oriented; contemporary nursing is more than a useful skill for a woman to have in the years between high school and marriage. The increase in the numbers of nurses who are heads of households and the changing role of women in American society have together contributed to the increased career orientation among nurses. Today's men and women demand more of nursing. They see nursing as a long-term involvement, an occupation within which they can develop and grow over a period of many years, experience personal fulfillment, and support a family.

Third, with the increasing professionalization of nursing has come the realization that more control over one's own practice is essential for full use of nursing expertise and to ensure that the nurse can remain true to professional commitment and respect the basic principles of ethics. Nursing education has changed so that nurses now expect control over their own practice and are increasingly prepared for more sophisticated duties and more independent judgment.

Although some of the newest trends in nursing have been toward more expert and autonomous positions, many of the positions that now exist still resemble the traditional subservient role of the hospital nurse of the 1950's. The image of nurses in the eye of the public does not always reflect the autonomy that nurses have begun to see as so important in their professional roles. The various social institutions that determine how nurses may practice have not been quick to change.

The nurse who seeks a job now receives conflicting signals both from within the profession and from society at large. Expected to be faithful in following orders, the nurse is accountable for independent, expert judgments. Expected to be a gentle caregiver for the sick, the nurse must also stand up assertively for professional principles. The perspective presented in this chapter is intended to assist the nurse in choosing a role while remaining faithful to that professional commitment.

THE DIVERSITY OF PRACTICE ROLES

The major changes in the health care delivery system that have taken place in the last 40 years have had a significant impact on the kinds of roles in which nurses now practice and on the roles that are likely to develop in the near future. In the decades prior to World War II most graduate nurses worked in the community; patients who could afford to do so often retained their own private duty nurses to care for them at home. These nurses contracted directly with patients for services rendered and fees paid. At that time the hospital staff nurse was not a highly skilled professional. Staff nurse positions were typically filled by nursing students as part of their training. In the late 1920's, 75 per cent of hospitals employed no graduate nurses in staff or general duty positions (Kalisch and Kalisch, 1975).

After World War II the hospital replaced the home as the center for acute care. Private duty nursing in the home declined as a source of employment for nurses. The hospital nurse performed many of the same functions of both the private duty nurse and the unskilled nursing student. Her role included many non-nursing tasks such as scrubbing floors and maintaining equipment.

The nurse's relationship with patients, which had been essentially a one-to-one relationship in private duty nursing, was altered in the institutional context. Hospital administrators followed the model of industry in their efforts to make hospitals more cost-effective. Efficient production was assumed to require that each worker perform small tasks repetitively (Drucker, 1954). In industry this might involve a worker placing the same screw in a large number of automobiles, with no sense of responsibility for or vision of the automobile that emerged farther down the assembly line. In the hospital, the same model involved a nurse moving from patient to patient at the designated hour, performing her assigned task, whether it be taking temperatures, dispensing medication, or bathing patients.

Industry has since questioned this method of production, suspecting that it was inefficient and resulted in worker dissatisfaction. When this model of production was applied in the hospital, it became difficult for a patient to recognize any one nurse as "his" nurse; he could no longer demand from the nurse the loyalty that a client expects from a caregiver with whom he has entered into a contract. The nurse's responsibility was to her superiors for the performance of assigned tasks on a series of patients. In short, the structure of staff nursing roles in the hospital worked against the establishment of professional-client relationships of nurses with their patients.

Hospital nursing at that time did not offer a great variety of roles. Nurses who wished career and wage advancement had to aspire to management positions and a promotion that removed them from direct patient care. Little opportunity existed for combining career advancement and decision-making with direct patient contact.

During the twentieth century health care has begun reaping the fruits of the scientific method as it emerged in the eighteenth and nineteenth centuries. Dramatic changes followed breakthroughs such as the discovery of antibiotics and the introduction of sophisticated technology into critical care. Largely as a result of new knowledge, the average life span of Americans has increased from 47.3 years in 1900 to 62.9 years in 1940 to 73.8 years in 1980 (U.S. Senate Special Committee on Aging, 1982).

That is certainly good news, but it tells only part of the story. Our increased ability to *preserve life* does not always enable us to *restore health*; decreased mortality has created a population with a higher prevalence of chronic disease. Hospital patients tend to be older and sicker than they were 20 years ago, and they create a greater demand for more intensive hospital care. These trends have contributed to unprecedented increases in health care costs. In the attempt to control costs, length of hospitalization has often been reduced. The net result has been an older, sicker population, requiring more sophisticated hospital care, returning home sooner, and requiring more follow-up in the community.

The vast amount of available and useful medical information has become too much for any one physician to assimilate and use in his practice. The medical profession has responded to the explosion of knowledge and technology by specialization. By concentrating within a fairly narrow area of medicine a doctor can remain current in his ever-developing field. With specialization have come new diagnostic and treatment procedures. Transplants, fluoroscopic examinations, mechanical ventilation, and hemodialysis are just a few of the now-common procedures that were extraordinary or experimental 25 to 30 years ago. Such new approaches in medicine have created a need for technically skilled and knowledgeable assistants to manage machinery and carry out complicated medical regimens. Specialties such as respiratory therapy, physical therapy, radiological technology, and others have taken on the tasks demanded by these new procedures; but nurses, too, have taken on many of these tasks, and more formalized nursing roles have developed to reflect the new duties. Today there is a confusing array of new roles for which the nurse may choose to be educated.

Nurses may choose now to practice in a wide variety of settings. Acute care hospitals offer a variety of specialty settings such as critical care units, rehabilitation units, oncology units, and outpatient clinics. A nurse may also choose to practice in long-term care, occupational health, community health, schools, day care centers, and senior citizens centers.

Still, hospitals continue to be the single largest group of employers of nurses. In 1980, 67 per cent of all working nurses were on hospital payrolls. Their roles have changed considerably since the 1940's and 1950's. Today the nurse has additional practice choices that need not remove the expert practitioner from patient care. Nurses who serve as clinical specialists and as patient educators spend a major portion of their time with patients, as do nurses who practice as enterostomal therapists or as members of cardiac or pulmonary rehabilitation teams. Nurses are now filling roles in such diverse areas as infection control, intravenous therapy, diagnostic laboratory work, and utilization review or quality assurance.

The Hospital Staff Nurse. Although increasing numbers of nurses are selecting newer roles, 71.9 per cent of all hospital-employed nurses in 1980 still worked in staff nurse or general-duty positions (Aiken, 1982). Hospital staff nursing has undergone some changes since its emergence as the most common form of nursing employment. The staff nurse of today has more formal education than her counterpart of 30 years ago. The ratio of staff nurses with at least a baccalaureate degree to those with a diploma from a hospital program but with no degree has gradually grown. Among nurses between 25 and 29 years of age (the group most highly represented in staff nurse positions), the percentage with at least a baccalaureate degree rose from 19 per cent in 1972 to 30 per cent in 1978 (American Nurses' Association, 1978). Numerous specialty organizations for various sorts of hospital nursing now exist and provide and encourage continuing education for their members. Several states now require continuing education as a condition of active licensure.

The better-educated staff nurse of the 1980's has begun to exert more control over practice situations. When the hospital exemption from the Taft-Hartley Act was repealed in 1974, unionization of hospital nurses became common. Within one year, 200,000 of the nation's practicing RN's were represented by unions (Kalisch and Kalisch, 1986, p. 681). Contract negotiations by unionized nurses can be used to control conditions of practice, and nurses have used them for such matters as improved wages, representation on hospital committees, better nurse-patient ratios, and improved orientation programs. Control over practice, many nurses have realized, is essential for the fulfillment of the professional's promise to provide the best possible care to clients.

Primary Nursing. One result in the hospital of this concern for control over practice conditions is a re-examination and restructuring of hospital roles for nurses. The introduction of *primary nursing* in the 1970's created the potential for a major change in the practice of bedside nursing, using the greater education of nurses and their desire to control their own professional actions. Primary nursing places the major responsibility for an individual patient's nursing care decisions with one nurse (the primary nurse), who works with the patient from admission to discharge. Primary nurses establish a plan of care for patients, provide at least some of that care themselves, and direct and monitor the care given by others (associate nurses). In addition to providing total patient care, the primary nurse maintains major responsibility for the patient's nursing care 24 hours a day, much as the patient's primary physician does for medical care. Decisions about changes in nursing care are made through the primary nurse. The result is a continuity of nursing care that would be otherwise difficult to achieve.

Primary nursing alters the way in which nursing decisions are made. Under two common alternative models, functional and team nursing, the head nurse or team leader communicates with the physician and then communicates downward to the nurse who actually provides patient care. In both of these alternative models, the nurse who most directly cares for the patient is at least one step removed from the source of major decisions concerning the patient's nursing care, whether that source be the physician, head nurse, or team leader. Consequently, the patient, too, is removed from those who make decisions concerning his care. The more removed the patient is from those who make decisions concerning his care, the more difficult it is for the decision-makers to consider the patient's own goals, desires, and choices. Even if practitioners respect patient autonomy, they cannot preserve the patient's autonomy as easily or completely when information does not reach them.

In primary nursing, the nurse who plans, directs, and gives the patient's care communicates directly with the physician and is directly responsible to the physician for carrying out medical orders and for planning a course of nursing care to complement the patient's medical management. The primary nurse becomes the patient's nurse, in a way that can be more properly identified as a professional-client relationship. This does much to avoid the impersonality of a system in which most of the patient's direct contact is with those health care workers who are "just following orders." Primary nursing presents greater opportunity for the nurse to exercise judgment and to develop the kind of loyalty to clients that forms the ethical bond in any true professional-client relationship.

If primary nursing sounds more attractive because of its opportunities for a more professional practice, it also places greater demands on nurses. The primary nurse remains subject to stringent quality control standards and must deal with the need to coordinate nursing care with that provided and requested by the physician. When disagreements arise, the nurse bears the obligation to work with the physician to resolve them. The patient who understands the nature of primary nursing will *legitimately* expect from the nurse a level of expertise and professional advocacy that he might not expect from the traditional staff nurse. The primary nurse must be prepared with an education appropriate to this increased responsibility. This makes demands on the individual nurse. The nurse obviously must be adequately educated and have the necessary social skills to provide this sort of care. It also makes demands on the institutions that prepare, certify, and employ nurses. Moreover, it demands of other health professionals a form of shared decision-making for which not all have been properly trained.

It is difficult to assess how many hospitals have actually implemented primary nursing. Some hospitals that claim to have instituted primary nursing have actually begun a sort of "modular" or "modified" primary nursing that stops short of the 24-hour responsibility by the nurse for the duration of the hospitalization. In attempting to implement primary nursing, hospitals often encounter difficulties in finding nurses with the necessary level of expertise, in making adequate use of present staff, and in changing the attitudes of the physicians who must work with primary nurses. Primary nursing is not simply a different way of getting routine nursing care tasks completed. It is a philosophy that in many ways exemplifies fully professional nursing practiced in a hospital setting.

Primary nursing provides greater opportunity for the nurse to collaborate with the physician in patient care management. It allows the nurse the professional autonomy to direct the nursing care of a particular client. It demands professional accountability to the patient for the failures or flaws both in the nursing plan and in the execution of it.

The Clinical Specialist. Some nurses in hospitals are now working as clinical specialists. Clinical specialists are educationally prepared with a master's degree and advanced skills in a specific clinical area. They manage and direct the care of clients with complex nursing needs and act as a resource for the nursing staff. They may consult with the nursing staff to help them establish nursing care plans or may plan and direct the care. The clinical specialist ordinarily has a great deal of flexibility in scheduled hours and everyday activities but must remain available to clients and to the nursing staff as their needs arise. Often these specialists report directly to the nursing administrator.

The role of the clinical specialist is complicated by an ambiguity about expertise and credentials. The role initially developed from two distinct but simultaneous movements within nursing education and nursing practice. In the practice setting these roles were called "clinician" or "clinical expert." Nurses filled them on the basis of clinical experience and expertise rather than formal education (Anderson, 1966). At the same time universities began to prepare advanced clinical practitioners with master's degrees (Peplau, 1965). They were granted the title "clinical specialist." Because the two movements developed without adequate communication and cooperation, the terms "clinical specialist" and "clinician" have come to be used interchangeably. The roles have developed differently from one institution to another. Nurses may hold a common title but have widely varying qualifications and job responsibilities. This creates a certain latitude for the nurse who wishes to design a role but it also creates problems.

In a professional-client relationship, it is important that the client know what expertise is being offered to him. A professional-client relationship must begin with a fully informed consent to the relationship. Otherwise it begins by dehumanizing the one who is not informed. A profession's commitment is questionable unless it ensures that the individual practitioners have the qualifications necessary to provide the services that they claim to provide. The ambiguity of the role and preparation of the clinical specialist indicates a need for more careful coordination between the academic institutions in which nurses are prepared and the institutions in which they practice.

In spite of the confusion, the introduction of the clinical specialist role has had a major influence on diversification of nursing roles within the hospital. Today nurses may specialize in clinical areas such as oncology, rehabilitation, alcoholism, renal diseases, and critical care nursing, in addition to the long-standing clinical specialties of maternity, child health, and psychiatric/mental health nursing.

Other Hospital Roles. Nurses assume a number of roles in the hospital that do not involve them in direct patient care. Often a nurse will direct a hospital's infection control efforts or function in some other aspect of quality assurance. Recent economic changes have required hospitals to monitor carefully the lengths of stay and resource consumption of patients. Nurses typically function in this utilization review process. Such roles require some technical expertise on the part of the nurse as well as the ability to work closely with members of other health professions. Political good judgment is essential in such roles.

The Nurse in the Community. There have also been considerable changes in nursing's role in the community. One phenomenon is a sort of exodus of nurses from the hospital to the community. The longer nurses remain in practice, the more likely it is that they will work in the community rather than in a hospital position. In 1978 89 per cent of employed nurses below the age of 25 were working in hospitals, but only 55 per cent of employed nurses over 50 years old worked in hospitals. Older nurses are more heavily represented in community health, occupational health, school nursing, and nursing education than nurses under 30 years of age (U.S. Department of Health and Human Services, 1981).

Nurses who choose to work with the elderly have traditionally had practice in a nursing home or long-term care facility. Such opportunities continue to exist, but the growing number of elderly persons in American society has created an increased interest in the appropriateness of existing services. This has led to experiments with a variety of other care settings for the elderly. Alternative living situations enable the elderly to remain independent as long as possible while receiving an integrated set of social and health services. Nurses can play a key role in the integration of the services now offered in diverse settings that include adult day care centers, multiservice senior centers, and retirement communities in addition to the more traditional nursing home.

Many challenging opportunities now exist in community settings. Community health nurses may work through the established public health system, in a city or county health department. Often the nurse coordinates the services provided by numerous agencies, such as nutrition programs, services for handicapped children, and social welfare services. Nurses provide direct client care in the home and services such as health teaching and screening in schools and senior citizen centers.

Home health nursing is a rapidly expanding area of practice. Traditionally, nurses who work with a visiting nurses association spend a major portion of their time providing physical nursing care to chronically or terminally ill patients in their homes. These nurses often develop long-term relationships with patients and families and have the opportunity to provide a continuity of care that is not possible in the hospital setting.

Home health nursing in the 1980's has become more technical and episodic, primarily in response to changing policies in acute care institutions. The move by third party-payors to prospective reimbursement for hospital care has resulted in a shorter average length of stay. Patients often return home in need of some of the same services that were formerly provided within the hospital. The demand for home care of this nature has exceeded the capacity of existing agencies to provide it. Many new home health agencies have developed, frequently under the auspices of for-profit corporations.

The entry of for-profit corporations in health care has resulted in a variety of new approaches to health care delivery. Health maintenance organizations, neighborhood health centers, and emergency care centers all provide opportunities for nurses. The private sector provides additional employment for nurses in occupational health nursing, which frequently involves an expansion of responsibilities beyond traditional ones. The occupational health nurse is often required to have nurse-practitioner training and is responsible for conducting pre-employment and annual worker physical examinations and providing routine emergency care in collaboration with a physician. The occupational health nurse is often a key figure in a company's efforts to control the rising costs of the health care that it funds for its employees. In recent years occupational health departments have begun to emphasize health promotion in such activities as smoking cessation clinics, health education seminars, exercise programs, and health screening.

The Nurse Practitioner and Expanded Roles. In 1965 the University of Colorado introduced a nurse practitioner option in its master's degree program in nursing. This option was intended to expand the practice of the community health nurse with healthy children in community settings, but other social forces helped mold the role of the nurse practitioner in a way different from what they had planned. At about the same time, there was much concern about a shortage of physicians, especially in rural areas. This shortage was due in part to the increased specialization of physicians, which caused a reduction in the number of physicans available for primary health care. The nurse practitioner role was soon identified as a physician extender role. Nurse practitioners were utilized to enable the physician to care for more people; they filled in, doing medical work when the physician was unavailable. The original intent of the formulators of the program had been for it to provide expert, independent nursing care rather than to assist in medical care, but the distinction became blurred. As a result, nurse practitioners have often been viewed as doctor-substitutes.

In reality, they are not trained as doctors and have neither the expertise nor the legal right to do many of the things that patients have come to expect from their physicians. However, recent years have seen a liberalization of some of the legal constraints on the nurse practitioner. Some states allow her to have limited hospital admitting privileges and others have granted nurse practitioners the legal right to prescribe certain medications. By 1980 some form of prescriptive authority for nurse practitioners had been implemented in 13 states (Batey and Holland, 1983). In 1983 New Jersey extended to certain nurses working outside the hospital the right to pronounce death.

Nurse practitioners perform many of the same tasks that general practice physicians do. They conduct physical examinations, order routine laboratory work, and manage minor illnesses. But their education and expertise lie in the areas of total family assessment and intervention, health teaching, and providing the counseling and support that individuals need to adjust to health problems. The nurse practitioner's clientele includes individuals who need these kinds of services more than they need complex medical diagnosis and treatment. Well children, women experiencing normal pregnancy and birth, adults with chronic diseases, and adolescents with developmental crises are examples of the kinds of patients the nurse practitioner is prepared to care for. If these persons develop acute illnesses or complex problems requiring intensive medical intervention, the nurse practitioner refers them to a physician. Likewise, the physician refers to the nurse those clients whose primary need is for nursing care. The client thus receives the full benefit of the complementary expertise of both professions.

Some health maintenance organizations (HMO's) have recently begun using nurse practitioners as the first contact with professional health care. HMO's are prepaid, subscription services that provide all a person's health needs for a single subscription fee. They attempt to reduce the cost of health care by providing both wellness care and early intervention in the beginning of health problems.

Expanded Roles and Professional Boundaries. The fluidity of the boundaries between the roles of physicians and of nurses who are acting in expanded roles poses a number of difficulties. Although the problems are most obvious to nurse practitioners, they are present for other nurses who work at the edge of professional boundaries. First, this fluidity may create confusion for the patient; he may not know what he can legitimately expect from the nurse. The patient has both a legal and an ethical right to the knowledge that enables him to make his own decisions rationally. It is conceivable that a patient might be more inclined to accept nurses in unfamiliar roles if he does not know that they are nurses. This might enable the nurse to gain his trust in order to provide professional care. In fact, in a study of nurses working as independent practitioners in psychotherapeutic roles it was found that four of six subject nurses did not identify themselves to patients as nurses. One nurse in the study said:

> I will define myself as a nurse practitioner when it is useful for me to do so and it's not a professional asset at this point to do that (Benton, 1979).

There is a conflict of ethical values in such a situation, one that is similar to the medical student who allows patients to identify him as a doctor. Nurses who choose not to identify themselves as nurses may do this in order to bypass a patient's misunderstanding of nursing expertise. Such a stance may be paternalistic: it seeks to benefit the patient by withholding information from him. The paternalistic motive is not in itself evil; it comes from a desire to do good to others. However, it always involves attempting to do good to others by taking from them the autonomy of their own decisions. In this case autonomy is lost because the patient is denied the information about the professional who proposed to help him, information that might help him decide about his treatment. If the patient's reluctance to accept the care of a nurse is based on ignorance of her capabilities, deceiving him does nothing to clear up his ignorance. The professional relationship requires not only that the professional *get* the trust of the client but that the client freely enter into the trust relationship that creates the bond. *Getting* trust and *earning* trust are not always the same thing; the former can be accomplished through deception, but the latter is always based on honesty.

As were the psychiatric nurses in Benton's study, nurses in nontraditional roles may be hampered in their practice by a public image of nursing that has not kept pace with the change to more expert, independent roles. Those nurses are in key positions to change the image of nursing, but they can do so only by identifying themselves as nurses and demonstrating to society that nurses can be trusted to fill these different roles. The stereotypical public image of nursing continues to restrict expanded practice, yet the nurses who function in nontraditional and possibly more appealing and challenging roles are not visible enough *as nurses* to change the public's view of the profession.

Finally, the confusion between physician and nurse roles can lead to interprofessional turf battles. In the 1960's, when the concept of expanded roles became popular, there was a shortage of physicians. The medical community willingly delegated numerous responsibilities to nurses. Nurses viewed their changing roles as advanced nursing, but others viewed them as physician extenders. Some sources are now predicting that by 1990 there will be a physician glut in this country. The probable result is that physicians will want to regain for themselves medical duties relinquished to nurses during the period of shortage. Nurses who have functioned primarily as physician extenders will find themselves ousted from roles that they accepted to fill a temporary need but for which they were less educationally prepared than physicians.

Nurses' willingness to serve in any capacity that may be needed is an indication of the good will with which most nurses enter the profession.

However, it has the unfortunate side effect of causing nursing to be viewed as a sort of do-all discipline whose members fill in when the "real experts" are unavailable or in short supply. Without a clear perception of what nursing is, both clients and nurses themselves tend to perceive nurses as fill-ins. One result is that patients do not know what they may legitimately expect from someone who is called a nurse, and the professional-client relationship that nurses are now seeing as the heart of their professional ethics is not developed.

Resolution of the problems associated with changing roles will require a perception of the nature of nursing that is more than the occasional documents produced by nursing scholars. The articulation of what nursing is about is a massive research and public relations project for the profession. It is also an important project of conscience for each individual who professes the title "nurse."

CHANGING ROLES AND THE LEGAL FRAMEWORK

An occupation's professional status, as we have seen, depends in part on the commitment and expertise of those who belong to it. But it also depends on the way society perceives and deals with that occupation. First, if the members of a society do not recognize both the expertise and good faith of the practitioners and the necessity of their services, they will not enter into that special bond of a professional-client relationship.

Second, a profession depends upon the various features of the *legal system* of the society in which it exists. The legal system acknowledges and protects the special relations that it believes should exist when an occupational group is recognized as a profession. The legal system is thus used as a formal embodiment of the moral relations between professions and society. A personal ethic that has been accepted by a community or society becomes explicit and enforceable when it is embodied in law. Legal structures serve a purpose that is at least twofold: they ensure that those who practice a profession practice only in areas in which they are legitimately competent, and they provide redress when the professional does not meet (or is accused of not meeting) the standards established by the profession for the public welfare.

An examination of nursing roles would be incomplete without a look at the legal framework that surrounds it. A look at laws and regulations concerning nursing can provide a sort of gauge of society's thinking about nursing, its understanding of nurses' expertise, and the level of its acceptance of nursing's claim to professional status. It would be impossible here to give a complete account of nursing and the law. Laws differ from state to state, and the law is constantly undergoing revision through both legislation and courtroom interpretation. We can only give some indication of the directions that the law is taking in response to nursing's entry into expanded roles and examine how such laws influence nursing's professional commitment.

The *nurse practice act* that each state adopts to legitimize nursing practice within its boundaries provides some of the most important legislation relating to nursing practice. It specifies what will be considered within the rightful functions of the nurse practicing in that state. In some cases it specifies not only what functions nurses will perform but also what will be acceptable preparation and competence to be able to perform the functions of a nurse. Nurse practice acts directly control the practice of nursing. Throughout the 1970's and early 1980's nurse practice acts have served as the arena within which much of the process of expanding nursing has been carried out.

Prior to the early 1970's most states used some version of a statement issued by the ANA on the scope of nursing practice adopted in the 1950's. That statement drew a rather rigid line between *nursing* and *medical* practice by declaring that the practice of professional nursing should not include "acts of diagnosis or prescription of therapeutic or corrective measures" (ANA, 1955). But the terms "diagnosis" and "prescription" cover a broad range of activities both within and outside of health care and do not in ordinary language describe only what physicians do. A *diagnosis* is a conclusion or judgment about the nature of a situation, and a *prescription* is a recommendation for a course of action directed toward changing a situation. In the broadest sense of these terms, mechanics, television repairmen, and countless other workers diagnose and prescribe as part of their routine activities.

Many common nursing activities also are forms of diagnosis and prescription. When a patient refuses to look at or begin caring for a new colostomy, the nurse diagnoses that the patient is having difficulty adjusting to a change in body image. The prescription may be to confront the patient about his difficulty and provide appropriate teaching and emotional support. When a patient with an endotracheal tube begins coughing violently, the nurse diagnoses that bronchial secretions are obstructing the tube. The prescription is to perform tracheal suction. Nurses diagnose troublesome pressure areas on the bedridden patient's skin, the patient's ability to carry out personal hygiene, and the degree to which the new diabetic understands dietary exchange lists.

These judgments are all related to nursing measures and ordinarily would cause no debate concerning whose responsibility they are. However, referring to such judgments as "nursing diagnoses" has led to resistance from some physicians who interpret diagnosis in the narrow sense of medical judgments that are the sole responsibility of the physician.

Difficulties also arise when we try to establish legal boundaries between nursing diagnoses and medical diagnoses in areas such as critical care or normal birthing. In these areas the two disciplines are closely related, and in practice many functions and judgments overlap. In the 1970's, as nurses began seeking out expanded roles and educational institutions began preparing them for these roles, many states saw the need for some revisions in their practice acts: a conception of nursing that rigidly excluded nurses from all diagnostic and prescriptive activities was no longer adequate, if it ever had been. A study conducted in 1978 of all 50 states showed that states have come up with a variety of ways of dealing with expanded roles for nurses (Trandel-Korenchuk and Trandel-Korenchuk, 1978). At the time of the study all 50 state boards of nursing reported some activity in the attempt to deal with expanded roles.

Some states did not change the wording of their nurse practice acts but began instead to interpret them more broadly to allow for the variety of developing roles that exist in nursing practice. Others inserted phrases and clauses that were intended to dictate a broader interpretation. California and several other states chose to redefine the scope of nursing rather than to patch up their former nurse practice acts; they chose to make specific reference to the new nursing activities that would be considered within the scope of nursing practice. A section of the California law recognizes the existence of overlapping functions between physicians and nurses and attempts to provide for collaboration between the two disciplines. Another approach has been to carefully define nursing diagnosis and nursing treatment, as the New York statute has attempted (Trandel-Korenchuk and Trandel-Korenchuk, 1978).

Some states have referred the question of the scope of nursing practice to some administrative body within the state rather than specifying directly within their practice acts what new roles nurses will be entitled to perform. The body is usually a board of nursing or medicine or the two groups together. The nature of the administrative body that is charged with determining the boundaries of nursing practice is important for the future of nursing in that state, since it may provide leadership in future efforts to revise the practice act.

Whatever method the individual state chooses to use in dealing with the issue of the expansion of nursing into previously unfamiliar areas, this issue remains a matter of importance for nursing. The law must constantly strike a balance between two extremes. It must not unnecessarily limit the scope of nursing because of irrelevant considerations even if they have been traditional; to do so would be unfair to both the clients served and the members of the profession. Neither must it extend the scope of nursing beyond the skills that we can reasonably expect from a nurse or into an area of practice more suited to some other profession.

The practice acts of the states are one significant force in determining the scope of nursing practice. A second influence comes from the courts, which provide important retrospective judgments about nursing practice. These judgments affect not only those involved in the individual case adjudicated but the members of the profession in general by establishing interpretations and precedents that serve as legal guidance in future cases. The limits of nursing practice are sometimes tested in the courts when a nurse is accused of practicing beyond what the law permits.

For example, in Missouri two nurse practitioners who practiced in a family planning clinic were accused of practicing medicine without appropriate licensure. The nurses performed pelvic examinations and dispensed vaginal medicines and intrauterine devices according to protocols but without direct supervision by a physician. A circuit court judge ruled against the nurses. Later the Missouri Supreme Court vindicated them, noting that these actions did not violate the provisions of the Missouri Nurse Practice Act (*Sermchief v. Gonzalez*). This case illustrates how the courts function to interpret the law in a specific instance. The decision handed down in this case then serves as a guideline in other similar situations.

Just as important for the future professional standing and responsibilities of nursing are those kinds of cases in which the courts have ruled that the nurse does in fact have responsibilities that she may not have taken seriously. In one 1980 court case in Massachusetts, a woman visited a nurse practitioner at a community health clinic because of dysfunctional bleeding and a foul vaginal odor (*Gugino v. Harvard Community Health Plan et al.*). The patient had had a Dalkon shield in place for three years. (This contraceptive device had since been removed from the market because of unusually high rates of pelvic and uterine infection.) The patient was told by the nurse that she probably had a lower gastrointestinal flu and was told to douche with yogurt for the vaginal odor.

Subsequently another health care provider treated the patient, who required a total hysterectomy for multiple abscesses. The nurse practitioner apparently misdiagnosed as a result of her lack of knowledge of the dangers of the Dalkon shield. The court, in charging the nurse with negligence, recognized the increased expertise that the client has the right to expect of a nurse specialist.

The law has long held nurses responsible for independent judgment when they are engaged in nursing activities. In *Norton v. Argonaut Insurance Company*, for example, a court held that a nurse was liable for administering a prescribed medication when she should have known its inappropriateness. Still, a nurse is responsible for following the orders of a physician (*Toth v. Community Hospital at Glen Cove*). In the Massachusetts case, the court held that nurses who take on new roles also accept responsibility for acquiring and applying increased knowledge and expertise.

The courts have also begun realizing that the nursing profession as a group bears the responsibility of establishing standards of acceptable practice that will be observed by its members. In one recent court case in Michigan, a nurse anesthetist was sued by a patient who suffered cardiac arrest during a surgery for which she administered the anesthesia (*Whitney v. Day, M.D.*

and Hurley Hospital). The trial court instructed the jury that "a nurse-anesthetist possesses responsibilities greater than those possessed by an ordinary nurse and that these responsibilities lie in an area of expertise which is akin to the practice of medicine." When the court ruled, it recognized that the standard of care to be expected and recognized as quality care by a nurse-anesthetist would be measured by the standard "already historically established by other similarly specialized, educated and experienced nurse-anesthetists" (Regan, 1981).

In effect, this court clearly recognized the special competence of the nurse specialist. This is more than a legal declaration to other groups not to meddle with nursing, and to permit them to establish their own standards. The court signaled its intention to rely on the profession to establish standards of care. Nursing specialties were thereby implicitly recognized and identified as having significant professional and legal responsibilities, both individually and as a group.

Society's acknowledgment of expanded roles for nurses is moving cautiously. Nurses themselves bear the burden of convincing society that they have the expertise to function in ways that society had not previously allowed. Nurses as a group must articulate and maintain the standards of clinical care and professionalism in the new roles that society entrusts to them. The changes in role that nurses are finding available to them are something more than increased job opportunities; they carry with them increased ethical responsibilities for the individual nurse as well as for the profession collectively.

MAKING AN ETHICAL CHOICE

Entering a profession involves one in societal institutions whose goal is to serve the welfare of persons. Choosing how and where to serve involves one in surveying the environment and its social institutions in order to see how to convert this choice into action.

Today's nurses face the choice of a variety of roles and institutional settings, because of the position of nursing as an emerging profession. They may choose a role that offers more or less autonomy in practice and that demands more or less expertise. They may choose a setting that either helps or hinders their efforts to serve as an advocate for their clients. How nurses make this choice will determine how successfully they can act on their original intent to be of service in a professional way.

Because nursing is already identified as a specific occupation, the roles and actions that one takes when identifying oneself as a nurse take on an added social dimension. They in effect define for society what nursing is. Thus, nursing in society is the sum of the roles and actions of individual nurses. Each nurse therefore contributes at least indirectly to the identity of nursing itself, whether she chooses to or not. The extreme of assuming that individual nurses represent only themselves fails to consider the societal expectations that are legitimized by nursing's claim to professional status. Professional life has a social meaning and creates legitimate expectations or rights that depend on more than what the individual professional desires or intends. It is inconsistent to claim membership in a profession while choosing roles that are impotent and that minimize one's ability to serve as an advocate and make use of professional expertise. A poor choice of a role or of a practice setting while retaining the claim to professionalism can lead nurses to pledge more than they are able to or intend to deliver.

For Further Discussion

1. Examine the nurse practice act in the state in which you intend to practice. Does it define the scope of nursing or assign that function to an administrative body? How are some of the newer roles discussed in this chapter dealt with by your state? Are there any changes that have been made recently or that are under consideration? How do these affect practice roles in your state?

2. Research recent literature to discover more about "nursing diagnoses." What issues are currently under discussion?

3. In many professional relationships, individual clients are free to choose their own professionals. This is commonly true of physicians, attorneys, and architects. Discuss whether (and how) it might be important for the individual to have such choices. How does it relate to the *ethical* bond created by an implicit contract between the professional and client? How does it relate to autonomy? When you have clarified ideas on this, examine nursing as a profession. How much choice do patients have in selecting the nurse who will care for them? If there is little or no choice, and if it is ethically important for the patient to have that kind of freedom, how can nurses compensate for that problem in their own direct dealings with patients?

4. List two or three roles in nursing in which you might like to practice. Then, find out what further opportunities there are to develop your expertise in these roles, e.g., journals, advanced study programs, continuing education, certification, specialty organizations. Using the definition of a profession developed in Chapter 1, assess to what degree a person might be able to practice nursing professionally in each role. You may wish to talk with someone currently practicing in each role.

Bibliography

Aiken, L. H. (editor) (1982). Nursing in the 1980's: Crises, Opportunities, Challenges. Philadelphia: J. B. Lippincott Company.

American Nurses' Association (1955). Suggestions for Major Provisions to Be Included in a Nursing Practice Act. New York: The Association.

American Nurses' Association (1981). Inventory of Registered Nurses, 1977-78. Kansas City, Missouri: The Association.

Anderson, L. C. (1966). The Clinical Nurse Expert. Nursing Outlook, 14(7):62.
Batey, M. V. and Holland, J. M. (1983). Impact of Structural Autonomy Accorded Through State Regulatory Policies on Nurses' Prescribing Practices. Image, 15(3):84.
Benton, D. W. (1979). You Want to Be a What? Nursing Outlook, 27(6):388.
Care, N. S. (1984). Career Choice. Ethics, 94(2):283-302.
Drucker, P. (1954). The Practice of Management. New York: Harper and Row.
Emmet, D. (1975). Rules, Roles and Relations. Boston: Beacon Press.
Ford, L. C. (1982). Nurse Practitioners: History of a New Idea and Predictions for the Future. In Aiken, L. H.: Nursing in the 1980's: Crises, Opportunities, and Challenges.
Fortin, J. D. and Rabinow, J. (1979). Legal Implications of Nursing Diagnosis. Nursing Clinics of North America, 14(553).
Gordon, M. (1982). Nursing Diagnosis: Process and Application. New York: McGraw-Hill.
Jones, P. E. (1979). A Terminology for Nursing Diagnoses. Advances in Nursing Science, 2(1):65.
Kalisch, B. and Kalisch, P. (1975). Slaves, Servants, or Saints? An Analysis of the System of Nurse Training in the United States, 1873-1948. Nursing Forum, 14(3):226.
Kalisch, B. and Kalisch, P. (1986). The Advance of American Nursing. Boston: Little, Brown, and Company.
Kim, M. J., McFarland, G. K. and McLane, A. M. (1984). Classification of Nursing Diagnoses: Proceedings of the Fifth National Conference. St. Louis: C.V. Mosby Company.
Peplau, H. (1965). Specialization in Professional Nursing. Nursing Service, 3:268.
Regan, A. (1981). Nurse-Specialists: Malpractice Targets—1981. Regan Report on Nursing Law, 21(11):1.
Trandel-Korenchuk, D. M. and Trandel-Korenchuk, K. M. (1978). How State Laws Recognize Advanced Nursing Practice. Nursing Outlook, November, 713.
United States Senate, Special Committee on Aging (1982). Developments in Aging: 1981: Part I. Washington, D.C.: United States Government Printing Office.

Chapter Six

THE NURSE AND OTHER PROFESSIONALS

Jolene Tuma was a clinical nursing instructor at the College of Southern Idaho in March of 1976. Her duties included performing nursing services while supervising student nurses at the Twin Falls Clinic and Hospital. Mrs. A., who had had leukemia for 12 years, was a patient at Twin Falls Hospital. At this admission, Mrs. A.'s doctor had told her that she was dying and that chemotherapy was her only hope for survival. He discussed the chemotherapeutic drugs with Mrs. A. and informed her of the side effects and risks involved in taking them. Nurse Tuma had asked to be assigned to care for Mrs. A. and to administer her chemotherapy.

When Nurse Tuma, accompanied by a student nurse, approached Mrs. A. to administer the drug, she noticed that Mrs. A. was crying. She told Nurse Tuma that she had controlled her leukemia for 12 years with natural foods and felt that God would perform a miracle for her. Nurse Tuma discussed alternate forms of cancer treatment with Mrs. A., such as therapeutic touch, laetril, and nutritional therapy. She explained to Mrs. A. that these therapies were not sanctioned by the medical profession. At Mrs. A.'s request, she agreed to return later that evening to continue the discussion with Mrs. A.'s family present. On leaving the room, Nurse Tuma asked the student to forget what she had witnessed because what she was doing "may not be ethical or legal."

That evening Nurse Tuma returned and continued the discussion with Mrs. A.'s family. She asked that they not inform the physician of their discussion. Mrs. A.'s son notified the physician of what had taken place.

The physician discontinued the chemotherapy but resumed it after further discussions between Mrs. A. and her family. Mrs. A. died two weeks later.

The physician complained to the hospital and subsequently to the Idaho Board of Nursing that Nurse Tuma had interfered with the doctor-patient relationship. The Board of Nursing moved to suspend Nurse Tuma's license for six months because of unprofessional conduct. The Supreme Court of Idaho overruled the decision, noting that unprofessional conduct was not adequately defined by the existing nurse practice act.

The case of Jolene Tuma is a true one, and it has received widespread attention in the nursing literature (Lewis, 1977; Gargaro, 1978a and b; Stanley, 1979, 1982). Typically, writers have analyzed the case in terms of the issue of informed consent. But the Tuma case involved a second important ethical issue that has received less attention in the nursing literature. It is an instance of what can happen when the health professions do not or cannot work together.

The subject of this chapter is the problem of nurses working together with other health care professionals. The professional interrelationship most troublesome to the nurse is the one with the physician, so we shall single it out for special attention. We will look briefly at the issue of informed consent in the Tuma case but will focus more specifically on the relationship between the nurse and the physician and the implications for the patient involved.

The ways in which doctors and nurses typically relate to each other create problems of various sorts that result in ethical dilemmas. The commonly proposed alternative of a team, when taken very literally, seems to advocate both a sound set of interprofessional relationships and maximum respect for the autonomy of the patient. But, as we shall see, a team approach creates problems of its own. The dilemma of how to structure the relationships among the various health professions will remain. However, our examination here will at least make clear what any proposed solution will have to take into consideration.

INFORMED CONSENT

The requirement of informed consent is a legal protection of a person's moral right to personal autonomy. The signing of a consent form should indicate that the patient has made an informed and free decision to undergo the procedure or treatment. Put very simply, a decision is informed if the person has all the information that he or she might consider helpful in reaching a decision and understands the information that is given. A decision is free when it is made without pressure or coercion from others. If there is some doubt concerning whether the patient has been given adequate information or is able to understand that information or if the patient is being coerced or pressured in any way, then the patient very likely has not made a free and informed decision. This would be true even if the legal signature has been obtained.

Meeting the criteria of an informed and free decision is difficult in health care settings, because of the complexity of treatment procedures and the dependent role of the patient in relation to those who are asking for consent. It is impossible to deal with the issue thoroughly in this text. Many good resources are available that discuss in depth the complexities of informed consent for medical care (Annas, 1978; Beauchamp and Childress, 1979; Cassileth *et al*, 1980; Davis and Aroskar, 1983; Holder, 1977; Langham, 1979; Roth *et al*, 1977; Siegler, 1977; Tait and Winslow, 1977). Study of this literature is important for nurses to aid them in acting ethically in situations involving patients' informed consent.

In the case described, the legal requirements for an informed consent had been fulfilled. But Nurse Tuma judged that Mrs. A. did not seem adequately prepared for the chemotherapy. Nurse Tuma was legitimately concerned that the patient had not given her fully informed consent for the chemotherapy. Because Nurse Tuma had some doubt about Mrs. A.'s consent, intervention was appropriate. To have proceeded without at least clarifying the situation may have violated Mrs. A.'s right to exert control over her own life. If Nurse Tuma had administered the chemotherapy while ignoring the patient's doubts and concerns, she would in effect be regarding her task as more important than the person she treated. As a matter of ordinary ethics, this would be wrong. As a matter of professional ethics, it becomes an even more important issue. The professional, as we saw in Chapter 3, has more than a duty to respect others as persons; he or she must also be an advocate. An advocate must take positive steps to restore another person's autonomy when it is threatened or diminished.

But we have also noted in previous chapters that the professional practices in a social context. When deciding how to intervene, the nurse must consider not just the one-to-one relationship with the client but numerous other aspects of the situation. One important consideration is the patient's relationships with other professionals, who also consider advocacy to be a part of their commitment to the patient. Members of the various professions all seek the autonomy that would permit them to meet their commitment without interference by others. In seeking to act as an advocate, the nurse must work with these other practitioners in ways that will not jeopardize their professional relationships with the patient. In the Tuma case, the nurse's actions may have been motivated by her desire to serve as the patient's advocate. However, they were interpreted by the physician as interfering with his relationship with the patient.

THE NURSE AND THE PHYSICIAN

The physician and the nurse must work closely together, often providing services simultaneously. The patient does not typically make an exclusive choice of either nursing care or medical care; he receives both simultaneously in what is supposed to be a coordinated plan of care. When mutual respect and open and clear communication between doctors and nurses is lost, that carefully coordinated care cannot be given to the patient. The case of Jolene Tuma's patient is ample demonstration of the result of mistrust and noncommunication between the professions.

Nurse Tuma, for whatever reasons, did not communicate directly to the physician her concern that the patient did not have all the information she wanted before consenting to chemotherapy. Instead, Nurse Tuma met secretly with the patient and her family, asking them not to report their meeting to the physician. As a result, the patient and her family were forced to choose between a good faith relationship with the nurse and one with the physician. In effect, they were presented with an exclusive choice between professional nursing care and professional medical care. The case is morally distressing because patients should not have to make such a choice; they are entitled to both medical and nursing care (as well as the unique forms of care provided by the other health care professions).

To practice ethically, nurses and physicians must examine the state of affairs that encourages mistrust and noncommunication and take the necessary steps to change it. There are strategies the individual nurse can employ to encourage the melding of nursing with medical care. There are also more fundamental social factors that push the resolution of such difficult ethical problems beyond the scope of the individual nurse acting only in a specific clinical situation. Influencing these factors requires long-term collective efforts of the profession as a whole. Once again we come up against the interface of professional issues with a truly professional clinical practice of nursing. The ability to fulfill one's commitment to the individual client requires an understanding of these larger issues and a willingness to work with others to address them.

Doctor-Nurse Communication

The failure of the physician and the nurse in the Tuma case to communicate openly and directly with each other is symptomatic of long-standing communication difficulties between the two professions. Sociologist Leonard Stein observed a pattern of communication between physicians and nurses that he called the "doctor-nurse game." The object of the game was for the nurse to take significant responsibility for decisions concerning patient care while giving the appearance of being passive. The physician sought the nurse's advice, but did it in such a way that neither party had to openly acknowledge to the other or to anyone observing the game that they were doing so. When both parties played the game well, both were considered winners. The unit ran smoothly and both the nurse and the physician appeared competent and efficient. If one or the other did not play the game or played it poorly, conflict arose and neither player looked his or her best (Stein, 1967).

Although Stein's observations were made nearly 20 years ago, they could have been made today. Too often even highly skilled nursing specialists defer to the physician rather than openly acknowledge their own patient care decisions. Nurses still tend to adopt passive behaviors in relation to physicians, and the latter continue to resist collaborative arrangements between the two professions (Russo, 1980; Lee, 1979a).

Doctor-nurse communication games are functional: they ensure the quality of patient care by enabling nursing expertise to be used in an environment that does not explicitly acknowledge the existence and value of nursing expertise. They are built upon a deception: those who play the games deceive themselves, each other, and the persons for whom the games are played. The deception prevents the development of a truly collaborative professional approach to patient care management, because it does not openly acknowledge the contributions that each of the professionals makes to the care of the patient.

The ultimate loser in these games is the patient. The patient's partnership in his own care is the most fundamental way of protecting his autonomy. But he cannot become a partner in his care if he does not know the true locus of recommendations and decision-making. One of the objects of the doctor-nurse game described by Stein was to disguise the true source of the nurse's recommendations. Thus, by design, these games keep from the patient information that he needs and obstruct his exercise of autonomy. To include the patient in decision-making requires clear and open communication among all members of the health team.

The patient loses in yet another way when doctors and nurses continue to play deceptive communication games. As long as caregivers exert energies to maintain a facade that perpetuates a stereotype, those energies are not used to the direct benefit of the patient. A collaborative relationship between the doctor and the nurse should promote the patient's best interests rather than place constraints upon the professionals caring for those interests. It is not just the nurse who is constrained in doctor-nurse games. The physician, too, is required to minimize the contribution of the nurse; he is prevented from accepting her as a useful resource until he completes the ritual of making her expertise appear to be his own. The input from the nurse, when it cannot successfully be incorporated into the doctor-nurse game, is relegated to a sort of limbo, with no assurance that it will ever emerge to aid the patient.

In short, poor communication between nurses and physicians perpetuates a stereotype of the omniscient physician and the submissive nurse with no expertise of her own. In doing so, it wastes valuable energy, obstructs open communication, and ultimately threatens the right of the patient to remain autonomous and be respected as a person. The games are played with a good purpose, to ensure that the nurse's expertise is used by the physician. They could even be viewed as constructive and creative survival techniques developed by nurses as a way of coping with institutional constraints that would otherwise prevent them from using their expertise for the good of the patients. But the disturbing question remains as to why these games must be played in order for patients to benefit from the expertise of both physicians and nurses.

A partial answer to the question lies in the perceived need among professionals and clients alike to make the physician appear to be the source of all health care decisions. Over the last century, because of a number of complex social and historical forces, Americans have granted their physicians unprecedented control over their health (Starr, 1982). The realities of today's complex health care delivery system suggest that responsibility for the patient's well-being is shared by a number of care providers. But the myth persists that the physician has absolute command over all aspects of care.

Medical Power

Medicine in American society has traditionally occupied the position of gatekeeper. It serves as the almost exclusive entry point for the typical patient into the health care system, and it serves as an overseer for the other health professions and for institutions such as hospitals. With a few recent exceptions, physicians are the only professional group with authority to admit and discharge patients from the nation's hospitals. Although there is a very gradual and modest movement toward practice without physician referral among other health professions, a physician's signature still must accompany nearly all requests for diagnostic studies, patient treatments, and medications.

Most third-party payors still require authorization by a physician before they will reimburse for care delivered by the other health professions. Third-party payors such as private insurance companies and government-controlled health care programs such as Medicaid and Medicare accounted for two thirds of health care payments in this country in 1979. Thus, physicians have both the legislative fiat and economic force to ensure that they are almost the exclusive entry point into the health care system.

The role of the physician in the hospital's economic survival gives him another sort of power over health care delivery. The medical staff usually possesses little formal authority over the administration of a hospital; it has traditionally acted in an advisory capacity to the hospital administrator. The physician can nevertheless exercise great informal control over the operations of a hospital because he controls the source of the hospital's revenue—patient admissions and treatments. As the number of physicians increases, it is becoming more common for physicians to offer services that compete directly with those offered by the hospitals, such as outpatient surgery centers, sophisticated in-office diagnostic activity, and urgent care-centers. Insurance companies and other third-party payors have gradually come to realize that minimizing hospital time for patients is cost effective for them, too; they have adjusted their policies to encourage these services offered by physicians. Consequently the physician is now both the primary market for and the primary competition to hospital care. The combination is a strong informal source of power.

The physician functions outside the hospital hierarchy. The medical staff of the hospital serves in an advisory capacity to the hospital administrator, but the physician's economic power makes it difficult for administrators to ignore that advice. The physician either has direct access to the hospital administrator or needs only to go through the chief of the medical staff to influence decision-making. If serious conflicts arise, a physician may lose admitting privileges, but hospitals are reluctant to take this step because the physician will take his patients with him.

The nurse, on the other hand, functions at the bottom of the organizational structure. In some hospitals the nurse who provides direct patient care may be as many as four levels away from the top nursing administrator in the organizational structure. To initiate changes or to voice a complaint, the nurse must work through the chain of command, addressing the team leader (if one exists), then the head nurse, the supervisor or clinical coordinator, and finally the nursing administrator or assistant administrator. Nurses are employees of the hospital; if they are involved in a conflict they realistically must face the possibility of losing their jobs. The hospital loses an employee but no significant source of revenue.

In very practical terms, the outcome of a disagreement or conflict between a nurse and a physician concerning patient care is heavily weighted in favor of the physician. Opinions and judgments of the two professional groups are not likely to be given equal consideration when conflicts must be settled by representatives of hospital administration. This imbalance of power between medicine and nursing may partially explain Nurse Tuma's actions in choosing not to use ordinary channels to resolve her concerns about the patient's lack of information. The physician involved in the Tuma case was part owner of the clinic in which the conflict took place. Thus he was not only a partner in the conflict but, as part of administration, was also in a position to decide how the conflict should be resolved.

Health care has become so complex that a physician cannot assume full responsibility even if he wields the potential power and authority to do so. Nurses and other caregivers have accepted much responsibility for the day-to-day management of patient care. The physician spends only a brief period of time with the hospitalized patient each day. He cannot oversee and accept responsibility for such activities as routine skin and wound care, adjustment of patient routines, and patient teaching.

Despite the realities, the myth that the physician actually oversees and controls all patient care is still prevalent. One recent survey showed that, of non-nursing, nonmedical respondents, 65 per cent believed that a nurse required a physician's orders to care for bedsores. Nearly 20 per cent believed that a nurse always needed a doctor's order to change bandages (Lee, 1979b). Both of these are routine forms of nursing care, subject to the judgment of the nurse, yet clients attributed the responsibility and authority for these interventions to the physician.

The physician's power and authority relative to the nurse is an extreme example of the imbalance of power between physicians and other health providers. The social power enjoyed by the physician as physician is enhanced in the doctor-nurse relationship by the fact that most physicians are male and most nurses are female. Similarly, nurses tend to be younger than physicians and have less education. These three factors—sex, age, and education—are all sources of social power in our society. In physician-nurse encounters these factors serve to reinforce the authoritativeness of the physician and put the nurse at a disadvantage regardless of the validity and usefulness of what she may have to contribute to the situation.

Sex Role Differences

During the first half of the twentieth century, the proportion of medical school admissions that were women was approximately 5 per cent. By 1980, the figure had grown to slightly more than 23 per cent (Mussacchio and Hough, 1981; Starr, 1982). The percentage of males in nursing was less than 1 per cent prior to 1966 and increased to nearly 3 per cent in 1980 (Aiken, 1982). Thus, in spite of modest changes during recent years, medicine and nursing remain divided as essentially male and female occupational groups.

In groups that are sharply defined along gender lines, group relationships tend to reflect general social expectations of male and female roles. The character of professional relationships between physicians and nurses is determined to a large extent by the socialization of the sexes in our society. Professional interactions often reflect traditional norms concerning male and female behavior.

Traditionally, nursing has been viewed as an occupation that was consistent with the feminine image. In fact, it embodied many of those characteristics associated with the ultimate, natural female role of mother. The good woman (and the good nurse) was caring, nurturing, expressive, and dependent upon the stronger, more aggressive male.

Medicine, on the other hand, embodied those characteristics valued in the traditional American male. The physician aggressively confronted disease and solved patients' health problems. He could be depended upon to take charge of the situation, act decisively, and tell others what needed to be done.

The re-emergence of the women's movement in the 1960's did much to change long-standing stereotypes of male and female roles. Being career-oriented and ambitious are behaviors no longer reinforced only in boys. Great strides have been made in liberating both men and women to develop fully as human beings and to pursue careers without the restrictions of sex-role stereotypes. Increasing numbers of women are now combining careers with families, and sex barriers in certain occupations are slowly disappearing.

These changes are gradually being reflected in nursing and medicine. Nurses as a group seem more career-oriented, as evidenced by greater numbers of nurses working and more nurses choosing full-time employment over part-time (Aiken, 1982). The increased specialization on the part of nurses and the move toward increased education can be seen as efforts to carve out a more secure career for themselves. As pointed out, more men are entering nursing and more women are entering medicine, making the gender distinction between the two professions less severe.

In spite of these advances toward less rigid sex-role expectations, the effects of traditional socialization are still a major influence on the manner in which doctors and nurses relate to one another. Many of the students entering these professions in the 1980's are heirs to early childhood socialization that occurred prior to the changes of the 1960's and 1970's. Studies of the sex-role orientation of college-age females indicate that young women entering nursing still identify more strongly with traditional female social roles than do women entering other fields, although differences between nursing students and non-nursing students have become less pronounced in recent years (Mulenkamp and Parsons, 1972; Meleis and Dagenais, 1981; Sprunck, 1980). The women entering nursing continue to associate nursing with traditional female roles. The professional socialization of these students is guided by nursing educators and practitioners who themselves are attempting to reconcile their own socialization as traditional women and as traditional nurses with the demands of new professional roles.

Likewise, 90 per cent of the practicing physicians of the 1980's are men who were also socialized prior to the "liberation" of the 1960's. These individuals were prepared to fill traditional male roles and interrelate with traditional females. As medical students, they have learned that the physician's role in relation to the nurse is one of dominance (Rein, 1977).

Thus, in spite of the social movement toward less rigid role definitions for men and women, the men of medicine and the women of nursing enter professional relationships with expectations born of long-standing socialization. Most often these expectations place the two groups in a dominant-submissive relationship rather than one of professional equals.

Educational Differences

Educational differences between physicians and nurses also perpetuate the imbalance of power between the two professions. The education of nurses and physicians differs both in the amount of formal education held by practitioners in the two fields, and in the manner in which the educational process is conducted. We will take a close look at nursing education itself later. For the present our discussion of education is primarily comparative in the context of interprofessional relationships.

The amount of formal educational preparation held by most nurses is much less than that held by the typical physician. All physicians have a minimum of eight years of postsecondary education within the university network. By the time a residency is completed, a practicing physician ordinarily has ten or more years of formal education beyond high school. The move toward specialization can make the physician's training even longer.

This is in stark contrast to the two or three years of technical education received by the majority of nurses. In 1980 72 per cent of all registered nurses had an associate degree or a diploma from a hospital-based program as their highest level of education. The number of nurses with Master's degrees increased fourfold from 1960 to 1980, but nurses with advanced (Master's or Doctoral) degrees still comprised only 4 per cent of all licensed nurses in 1978 (ANA, 1981). Thus only a very small percentage of nurses have formal education comparable in length to that held by most physicians.

The discrepancy in educational preparation is a function of the lack of consensus within the nursing profession about what constitutes minimal requirements for entry into practice. The confusion about educational requirements has resulted in nurses with various levels of preparation functioning in essentially the same roles. Thus, even highly educated and specialized nurses are not readily evident because of poorly defined practice roles.

The differences in length of formal education of nurses and physicians is problematic for at least two reasons. First, it is a recurrent theme in nursing that nursing expertise is *different from* but *equal to* that of medicine. Although nurses have correctly stated that nursing skills are unique and different from medical skills, differences are not enough to guarantee their equality. Physicians and nonphysicians alike will inevitably compare the two groups and question the equality of expertise in light of such large educational differences.

A second problem that accompanies these educational discrepancies between physicians and nurses concerns those few nurses who presently possess advanced educational credentials. These nurses with advanced preparation bear the burden of distinguishing themselves from all other nurses. With so many different levels of preparation among nurses (many of whom appear to be doing the same thing regardless of educational background) it is understandable that physicians will not automatically accept all nurses as peers. One value of doctor-nurse communication games is that they provide a way for physicians to make use of nursing expertise when and where they find it without having to formally acknowledge all nurses as professional equals. Although this approach may ensure that nursing expertise is being used to the patients' benefit, it creates the problems of respect for patient autonomy discussed already. In addition, it prevents those nurses with appropriate credentials from being accepted as legitimate professional peers by their colleagues in medicine. The most expert nurses remain somewhat invisible to the clients, and the social influence, esteem, and compensation that accompany advanced education are reserved for the physician.

Differences in the *manner* of education are as important as differences in the amount of education when we try to understand the power relationships that exist between physicians and nurses. Young physicians learn early that they are fully responsible for the patient's welfare. They must be decisive and aggressive in diagnosing and treating disease. They are encouraged to accept responsibility for mistakes and must live with the knowledge that their mistakes can be fatal. One author describes the "Captain Medicine" mentality that medical students develop when they first begin to function in clinical situations:

> Early in the student's education. . . . the image of the house officer emerges vividly. He is the exhausted yet somehow dashing figure toting a bellboy and dressed in surgical greens. He is the one who knows just what to do when that disastrous motorcycle accident is brought into the emergency room. He starts the IV, gives the bicarb. He administers the cardiac massage. It is he who seems comfortable with the catastrophic, overwhelming and unimaginable. . . . Always, the student remembers that it is this figure whom the student will become in just a few short years (Resser and Schroder, 1980).

The young physician is socialized to take control of situations and lead patient care efforts. Other health professionals are viewed as assistants, ready to serve him in his work (Stein, 1967; Kalisch, 1975).

Student nurses, on the other hand, have traditionally been socialized for much less dominant roles. The historical roots of nursing education lie not in the university environment, but in military and religiously affiliated hospital schools of nursing. Traditional educational programs enforced rigid schedules and codes of conduct. Following orders and assisting the physician were major aspects of the nurse's role. As a women's profession, nursing exemplified traditional female roles of passiveness and dependence.

Although nursing education in the 1980's is dramatically different from that of the early part of the century, old traditions die slowly. Critics of contemporary educational practices charge that remnants of outdated socialization practices persist. Some nursing programs still enforce stringent dormitory rules, highly regimented schedules, and faculty intrusion into the nonclassroom behaviors of students (Cohen, 1981).

Student-faculty relationships in nursing education sometimes work at cross-purposes with the professional requirement for independent behaviors. The instructor may hover over students, often assuming a surrogate mother role. The instructor supervises and nurtures the student at the same time (Cohen, 1981). Unlike the young physician who is encouraged to accept the responsibility for the patient's well-being and learn to deal with the emotional burden of potential errors in judgment, young nurses are socialized to rely on others to provide direction and protect them and their patients from errors.

Age Differences

In the hospital setting, where the bulk of nurse-physician interactions occur, the majority of nurses (approximately 87 per cent) are under 25 years of age (ANA, 1981). Nearly 60 per cent of all practicing physicians are over 40 years of age (AMA, 1983). These age differences are in part attributable to differences in the length of time required for the educational program. A certain degree of social deference is associated with age. Age serves to elevate one in the eyes of others, particularly when it is accompanied by other elements of social esteem, such as money or position or sex.

In summary, the American physician is usually older, more highly educated, and more likely to be socialized to take control than is the typical nurse. The physician is in a powerful, dominant role, while the nurse is in a dependent, obedient role. Communication patterns within health care institutions reflect these roles, which in turn reflect male-female relationship patterns in society at large.

At least one writer has used the metaphor of a family to describe nurse-physician relationships within the hospital setting (Ashley, 1976). The physician is the hospital father, carrying out the role of the dominant decision-maker and breadwinner. The nurse has accepted the mother role; she follows the physician's orders, keeping the house in order during his absences. She acts as the primary caregiver and nurturer to the hospital children, the dependent and obedient patients.

The metaphor is apt, and it highlights the difficulties that nurses experience when they attempt to take a more decisive role in patient care. One difficulty is that nursing expertise is underappreciated. The very existence of doctor-nurse games provides testimony that the nurse's knowledge is in fact valued in health care. But it testifies at the same time that the nurse whose knowledge is valued is not openly recognized as being knowledgeable. Traditional sex roles and hospital structures are part of the reason for this, but so is the diversity of educational levels and expertise among different nurses.

The status of doctor-nurse relations is a quality of care issue. We have already noted that nursing expertise may sometimes be wasted if it must first be granted credibility by the physician before it can serve the patient. Quality of care issues are necessarily also ethical issues because of the professional commitment to provide an optimum level of care.

Among the more long-term effects of continuing to engage in deceptive communication games is the evaporation of the nurse's sense of self as a committed professional. Nurses who consistently pretend not to have expertise of their own may become comfortable with that position and begin to lose incentive to maintain standards of nursing care that patients deserve. Similarly, by pretending not to be the source of recommendations for patient care the nurse fails to cultivate the habit of accepting responsibility or at least will not adjust to it comfortably. The denial of responsibility can become a comfortable habit, one that is inconsistent with claims to professional status.

COLLABORATION

Fortunately, not all nurse-physician interactions conform to the deceptive game-playing encounters described by Stein. In fact, many nurses and physicians have worked together to redefine their roles in relation to each other. One major effort to address the problems of nurse-physician relationships was the development of the National Joint Practice Commission. This commission was established as a forum for representatives of both professions to examine the roles and functions of each, define new roles and relationships, and attempt to remove sources of differences in order that the two professions could work more in harmony with each other for the benefit of patients (ANA, 1981).

The kinds of relationships recommended by the Joint Practice Commission are based on a model of collaboration. Collaboration means working together toward a common goal, pooling the resources of both professionals in a mutually respectful and interdependent fashion so that the patient being served receives the full benefit of each provider's expertise.

In order for nurses and physicians to collaborate, certain conditions must exist (Alfano, 1981). First, the individuals must trust and respect each other as persons and as knowledgeable and competent professionals, each of whom has an important contribution to make to patient care. Second, they must have some core of common language, which allows them to talk with and understand each other. The third essential element of collaborative practice is shared responsibility and mutual or shared decision-making. Each professional offers suggestions based on knowledge and expertise that are incorporated into a mutual plan of care.

The Joint Practice Commission conducted model projects in joint or collaborative practice in four hospitals and developed recommendations and guidelines for establishing joint practice arrangements (ANA, 1981). The principles of collaboration underlying these joint practice guidelines can be applied in various settings. Some nurses and physicians have established joint practices in primary care settings, for example.

The efforts to facilitate joint practice have been at least partially successful in improving communication between the professions of medicine and nursing. The dialogue that has resulted from participation in state and local joint practice committees and other joint practice activities has increased understanding between the two professions and helped to resolve some of the turf battles between the two groups.

Dealing with Nurse-Physician Conflicts

Jolene Tuma evidently believed that this physician was not willing to work with her in a collaborative manner. We cannot decide here whether she was right or wrong in that belief. But the situation that she perceived herself to be in raises an important question: What should you do when all else fails in your efforts to work cooperatively with the physician, when you cannot agree with a patient care decision that you cannot change?

Mappes has proposed that you must first determine the nature of your objection—that is, whether you believe that the physician's orders are not in the best medical interests of the patient or whether you believe that they somehow violate the rights of the patient (Mappes, 1981). If the disagreement is about a medical judgment, then nurses must determine whether they have sufficient reason to rely on their own medical judgment rather than that of the physician. An honest evaluation of one's own expertise is essential here, but when an incident is so serious that a life is at stake, nurses ought to question an order even when less than certain of their own competence.

A nurse may sometimes disagree with a physician's order for reasons of ethics without questioning his medical judgment. The right of the patient to self-determination can be threatened even by a treatment that is medically acceptable. Here the matter is a bit different. Because physicians' medical expertise does not make them more qualified than nurses to make decisions on an ethical basis, there is no reason for nurses to defer to physicians' superior medical knowledge. Instead, nurses need to assess their own ability to think carefully about ethics.

Whether the reason for a nurse's disagreement with a physician's action is medical or moral, the nurse faces the uncomfortable issue of going through channels even when those channels are suspected to be ineffective. The Code for Nurses proposes that the nurse should first express concern directly to the "person carrying out the questionable practice" and call attention "to the possible detrimental effect upon the client's welfare"(ANA Code for Nurses, 1985, Item 3). If necessary the nurse should then go to appropriate authority within the institution. To do so, the individual must know the channels of communication within the institution and know how to use them properly, documenting all claims.

If the problem cannot be corrected within the employment setting, the code suggests that the nurse report the problem to other "appropriate professional organizations or the legally constituted bodies concerned with licensing." The code reminds nurses also of the right to refuse to participate in procedures to which they are personally opposed. But this should be done only if the refusal is made known in advance and in time for the institution to make other arrangements for the patient's nursing care.

The Code for Nurses offers this advice while attempting to observe three different, very important, ethical principles. The first is the patient's right to adequate treatment and to human respect. The second, which is derived from the first, is the necessity for preserving some sort of structure within the institution. As Mappes notes:

> Clearly, questioning at some point must cease. Otherwise, hospitals could not function efficiently and as a result the medical interests of all patients would suffer (Mappes,1981; p. 98).

Strategies used by the nurse in questioning medical orders must have the double and potentially conflicting goals of ensuring the welfare or rights of the individual patient and of preserving the kind of orderly system that provides for the welfare of all patients. Although the problem can be encapsulated in a formula, its solution cannot.

The third principle proposed in the code is the right of the nurse to refuse to participate in a procedure known or believed to be medically or ethically wrong. Here the code presents another sort of dilemma: withdrawing from a case has as its likely result only that the nurse who withdraws will not be the one to provide nursing services. It does not ensure that the services will not be provided. Before undertaking a conscientious refusal, nurses must ask themselves whether it is the violation of the patient's rights or welfare that motivates the refusal. If it is, then little is to be gained merely by refusing to participate and taking no further action. Jolene Tuma, for example, had to have realized that, if she simply refused to administer the chemotherapy, the ethical problem would not have been solved. Someone else would have been found to administer it in her place.

Nurse Tuma also faced problems related to the other two principles stated in the Code for Nurses. Her choice about what to do concerning the conflict between the patient's right to adequate treatment and the necessity for preserving structure within the institution is not so obviously correct. She chose a solution having ramifications that went beyond the immediate problem; the patient was left with no further possibility of receiving the services of both this dedicated nurse and the physician. To know whether there was another way in which Nurse Tuma could have protected her patient would require much more intimate knowledge of the situation than we observers can have.

THE NEED FOR A TEAM

The Jolene Tuma case offers a good example of what can happen when nurses and physicians fail to work together in the delivery of patient care. But nurse-physician collaboration resolves only some of the problems that exist in today's health care system. Efforts to improve working relationships between nurses and physicians ignore the reality that many providers, not just two, are important to meeting the needs of the whole person being served. Social workers, physical therapists, dietitians, psychologists, speech and hearing pathologists, occupational therapists, pharmacists, and clergy are only some of the professionals whose expertise is vital to the recovery or well-being of patients. Interprofessional relationships must develop in such a way that the contributions and expertise of all professionals will be maximized for the benefit of the patients being served. The concept of a team provides one possible form for that relationship.

It is not uncommon to hear health professionals make casual reference to the "health care team" when discussing other professionals with whom they work. Research has shown that, although health professionals may be very supportive of the team concept, they have different and sometimes contradictory ideas about what a team is (Temkin-Greener, 1983). The following discussion will look at the idea of team in its purest possible form. Teams of this sort might not actually exist or might not even be desirable. But the most extreme counterexample to interprofessional mistrust and noncooperation may help in deciding what kind of relationships are both ethically satisfactory and actually attainable.

The Concept of a Team

A team is a group of people who function as and are looked at as a single entity rather than simply a collection of individuals. A team has a shared goal that binds individual members together. Success is measured in terms of the team and achievement of the common goal, rather than in terms of the achievements of individuals on the team. A success for one member of a team is a success for the team. When it is possible for a member of the team to be a success while other members fail, there is no true team. On a sports team, for example, either the team wins or the team loses. It is impossible for some members of the team to win and others to lose.

For a health care team to have a shared goal, it must be able to transcend criteria of success dictated by individual professional specializations in order to arrive at a common criterion of success. This criterion should logically have something to do with the care of and needs of the patient. It may be the restoration or maintenance of health or function, but it may also be adjustment to permanent disability or even a comfortable death. The specific goals of the health team change to reflect the needs of the patient being served, and the team must adjust to such changes in common goals while providing their individual specialties.

Though a team has a shared goal, there are ordinarily differentiated functions within the team. The most reasonable way to differentiate functions on a health care team is through specialized expertise. However, care must be taken to ensure that the individual need being met by a specific professional's function is perceived in its relation to the client as a whole. Ducanis and Golin express it thus:

> Although the professionals may be expert in only a few aspects of the client's needs, they nevertheless must be concerned with all aspects of the client. Comprehensive care requires that the team deal with the client as a totality. This is not to say that the team will not emphasize one or another aspect of need at a particular time, but rather that no aspect of the client's problem should be neglected (The Interdisciplinary Health Care Team, 1979; p. 59).

Even though functions may be differentiated within a team, its cooperative activity toward a shared goal gives it the kind of unity that makes it more than a collection of individuals. But it is not yet a team unless the efforts that each member makes toward the accomplishment of the shared goal are designed and planned in cooperation with the efforts made by the other members. In short, a team is more than a group of individuals who have the same goal. It is a group of persons engaged in collaborative activity around a common goal.

The Team and Patient Autonomy

We noted in Chapter 3 that professionals have special duties to preserve or enhance the autonomy of their clients because the knowledge they possess can either threaten the autonomy of a vulnerable patient or support and enhance it. An unnecessarily paternalistic relationship does not respect the patient as a person because it does not treat him as a being with goals of his own and capable of making decisions of his own. Respect for the patient as a human being requires a relationship more like a contract between the professional and client, in which both become partners in meeting the client's needs. This model of the one-to-one professional-client relationship is ethically praiseworthy, but it does not reflect the reality of a society in which the knowledge explosion has resulted in specialization. No longer is one health professional responsible for satisfying all of the patient's needs. The stroke patient, to cite just one example, may find himself involved in various relationships with various different professionals, each of whom has a unique contribution to offer.

In a model of professional-client relationships which involves many professionals and one client, each professional relationship may well be beyond reproach when viewed in isolation from the others. In each discrete professional relationship, the patient is fully respected and regarded as an autonomous partner in a freely chosen relationship. But another problem emerges here. Note that the patient may still be regarded as divided. Although each professional sees him as a person, separating care according to specialties may still have the cumulative effect of separating the person into distinct and separate needs. When a person's psychological rehabilitation is separated from his physical rehabilitation from his nursing care and his medical management, that person becomes seen as a client with an individual problem by a series of individual professional practitioners. The danger is that the parts taken separately do not add up to the whole.

A person is not composed of discrete and distinctive needs; they are all unified in that person's experience. The demands of highly technical knowledge require that we make some effort to distinguish the various needs. What is also needed is some effort to reintegrate the person, to ensure that the efforts made by various professionals to satisfy individual needs are united by the wholeness of the person.

A person is an organic whole. His needs and skills, his decisions and goals are all interrelated in that person. Respect for persons requires that we treat them as wholes. Anything that the professional might do to fragment the unity of a person's life undermines his autonomy or self-determination. And this may happen even when each individual, specialized professional conscientiously treats the patient as a person within their own relationship. The stroke patient may regain maximum muscle and limb function through his professional relationship with the physical therapist. He may regain the ability to perform certain activities of daily living using assistive devices and techniques provided by the occupational therapist. Yet without proper psychological and social support, the patient may be unable to function independently because of an altered body image or overprotective behaviors on the part of his family. The stroke patient's maximum rehabilitation cannot be achieved unless all the individualized specialty care is provided in an integrated way to the total individual.

Where do we look for the thread to "hold the patient together" in the midst of professional specialization? It has sometimes been suggested that this is part of the nurse's function. The Social Policy Statement (ANA, 1982) seeks to describe the essence of nursing, by asserting the nurse's responsibility for reintegrating the patient's life in the face of major health changes. A similar view is developed by Sally Gadow, in her discussion of existential advocacy (Gadow, 1980). Indeed, this may very well be the ideal function of nursing.

There may be a discrepancy between the ideal function of nursing and nursing as it can be practiced within the world that now exists. Efforts to ensure that the patient is approached as a whole person must occur at two different levels. The threats to the unity of the patient as a person occur both within himself (because of changes in his body and alterations of body image) and external to him (because of factors in the caregiving situation). This would require that the nurse be able to address the patient and the patient's situation on both these levels, using various kinds of expert knowledge.

Given both the level of their own training as well as the way in which nursing as a profession is accepted in our society, it may be expecting too much of contemporary nurses to demand of them that they serve as the integrator of all care for the patient. Instead of being typically one of the least educated professionals, the nurse might have to be one of the most educated ones, incorporating into practice knowledge that is used by all of the other professions as well as knowledge to provide bedside nursing care. In addition, the nurse would have to function as a very special leader among health professionals and be recognized as such by them. This may well be an ideal worth pursuing for the future of nursing. It is not, however, an ideal that will easily or soon be achieved.

The problem then remains to find a way of integrating the care of the person in the present situation, a form of caring that can be given in the world as it now exists. This is when the implementation of a TEAM begins to appear important.

Delivery of health care through the team method has great potential for increasing respect for patients as persons by reducing the fragmentation caused by specialization. If each team member sees his or her contribution of a specialty as only one part of the general goal of care for the patient as a person, those specialties become reintegrated. But the process is more than an intellectual awareness of how the goal of the individual caregiver's service relates to some more general goal. It requires communication, so that each individual can see how his or her care continues to fit into the picture of a more general care for the total person, when the care and the person are dynamic and changing.

The Problem of Team Leadership

The health care team may well sound like a panacea, the end to all interprofessional problems in health care. In fact, it presents new difficulties both in its implementation and in its successful operation. Leadership is always a problem for teams. In preparing this book, when we discussed the issue of team leadership with one pediatrician, his response was: "Of course I believe in team care. But every team must have a captain and I am that captain."

Several things are worth noting about such a response. First, it in some ways reflects the realities of practice situations today; even the physician who is willing must, by law, continue to serve as a gatekeeper. But just as important is the physician's understanding of what it is to be a leader. To this physician, the leader is equivalent to a captain of a ship. Disagreements become like mutinies. This is a highly authoritarian model of leadership, one in which the leader uses positional and personal power to retain responsibility for all goal setting and decision-making and motivates subordinates by praise, blame, and reward. It is the kind of leadership that ensures that only one person must truly claim that "the buck stops here."

Leadership can take other forms as well. In essence, a leader is the person who facilitates achievement of group goals by influencing members of the group to organize their efforts toward the goal. The authoritarian model described is just one way of leading a group. The *participative leader* allows for varying degrees of participation by all members of the team. He or she may present an analysis of problems and proposals for action to the group. The leader then invites and considers comments and criticisms from all group members before a decision is made. The leader ultimately makes the decision and may choose to accept or reject suggestions from the team. In a group held together in this way, communication is encouraged, but lines of authority are carefully preserved.

A third model, *democratic leadership*, values the abilities and knowledge of each team member. The leader uses positional or personal power not to control and manipulate team members, but rather to draw out their ideas and motivate them to set group goals and decide how to achieve them. In democratic leadership, decisions are made by the team, not by its leaders. The leader facilitates the group decision-making process.

Which of these models of leadership is appropriate for any given group will depend on a variety of factors, including the personalities of the team members, their respective skills, the size of the team, the nature of their goals, and the environmental and time constraints under which they operate. To assume that an authoritarian model of leadership is the appropriate one is to unnecessarily limit the possibilities for teamwork.

A second feature of this one pediatrician's attitude toward leadership is important here: he assumes that the proper role of the physician is to be a leader. There may be many times in health care when this is appropriate. But if, as we have already argued, the goal of team care is the patient as person, and if the priority of specific needs is dependent upon the patient's own autonomous preferences, then there is good reason for thinking that both the manner of leadership and the decision of who should be the leader should be flexible enough to shift according to the changing needs and choices of the patient.

Whatever person or manner of leadership emerges as appropriate for the health care team, there is a world of difference between the respect that professional members of a team owe one another and the deference that leaders sometimes demand. If a physician turns out to be the most appropriate leader for a health care team, the recognition that he is a leader does not require the deferential behavior that nurses have traditionally shown physicians. Although some such deferential behaviors are becoming less common, they still remain in subtle ways. As recently as 1976, a nurse sociologist who studied the stratification system of a hospital nursing unit observed nurses standing when the physician entered the nursing station, pulling the physician's charts for him, carrying charts while making rounds with the physician, and speaking only upon receiving a cue from the physician. In contrast, physicians interrupted patient care, called nurses away from patients to do minor tasks, and praised nurses for solicitous behaviors toward physicians (Lewis, 1976).

Such behavior indicates that real impediments to team health care still exist in clinical practice settings. The rigid location of health care professionals into certain places in a professional hierarchy effectively prevents the operation of a team of equals. It just as effectively prevents the adjustment of care according to the needs of the patient, and this makes it an ethical issue that concerns the patient as a person. Respect is essential for a health care team; it involves the recognition that the other has a significant contribution to make. Deference, however, involves the explicit recognition of the lesser worth of one or more parties; it is incompatible with team health care.

These various issues in team leadership suggest that the issue of whether the physician should be a team leader is not exactly the heart of the matter. Style of leadership and the team environment as well as the ethical requirement of respecting the patient's goals for his own life all combine to complicate the question of leadership. To assume that team leadership is nothing more than another occasion for debate concerning physician dominance is to ignore some very important problems.

Teams and Collective Responsibility

The cohesiveness of the team makes it seem attractive, because unity facilitates communication and devotion to a single common goal. There is one puzzling consequence of a concept of team goals, decisions, and actions: the team begins to take on a character of its own, so that the team itself as a single entity becomes responsible for its actions. That we think in this way is manifest in our everyday language: we claim that our professional organizations do things, that hospitals make decisions, and that nursing schools have goals. The danger in thinking and speaking in such ways is that it can tempt us to think that the individuals who form the group no longer bear responsibility individually for what the team does or even for what they themselves do as members of the team. Ethics could easily disappear from health care if we managed to convince ourselves that, as long as we work as part of a group, we are not responsible as individuals for what we do. Philosophers have become quite interested in this problem for the last 15 years, and several of them have argued that we are not contradicting ourselves if we claim that both the team and its members are responsible for what a team does (see discussions in Ozar, 1982; Smith, 1982; and French, 1972).

Another phenomenon that can occur when we begin identifying with a team is called the "risky shift." Some studies indicate that persons in groups tend to make decisions that involve substantially more risk than they would permit in decisions that they make individually. There are a variety of explanations for this. It may be that the group provides the persuasion necessary for risk-taking. Or it may be that group involvement makes the individual feel less responsible and therefore more willing to take risks. Other views hold that group discussion makes those involved in the decision more familiar with the situation and thus more willing to take risks (Ducanis and Golin, 1979).

Team members should be aware of the risky shift phenomenon, as it may well affect the nature of the health care decision. This is true even under the optimal condition in which the patient himself can function as a member of the team caring for him. Forces other than the patient's own reasoning concerning his health care decisions may influence him to make decisions more risky than he would otherwise make. The team itself may function to hinder the patient's absolutely free consent. If that is the case, it is imperative that the team find some way to counteract its own hindering effect on free and informed consent.

The need to learn the art of team functioning has received inadequate attention in most professional curricula. To the individual, professionalization has usually meant the development of an identity within the profession rather than learning to function as a professional in cooperation with other professions. Students of the various health professions may have an understanding of teamwork or collaboration within a single profession but may not necessarily understand or agree about how members of the different professions can best work together. Students emerging into the world of practice are thus underprepared for assuming a position within a health care team, even if they emerge with expert individual skills.

Consensus building is important in teams. Teams without common goals and coordinated efforts are not really teams. For that reason, teams exert great effort in creating and maintaining themselves. The maintenance of the team can easily become the team's primary goal, replacing the goal for which the team was created. The shift in goals may not be noticeable until the team faces a situation in which the members disagree about the best course of action. If it becomes more important to avoid disagreement than to choose the best course of care for the patient, then the team loses its reason for existence. This is true for patient care teams, and it becomes true for other team efforts such as institutional ethics committees.

Devotion to teams and the team process can have another very disastrous effect. Knowing the worth of a team can lead one to adopt the rhetoric of team work and to pretend to be part of a team even in an environment that prevents real teams from developing. One author has described the effect in the hospital setting:

> Team talk seems to hide the real need for change in the hospital by suppressing feelings of alienation or by manipulating people to feel guilty, while the causes of alienation are allowed to continue (Erde, 1981).

In summary, team delivery of care seems to overcome some of the problems caused by the variety of professionals caring for the same patient. But teamwork requires a supportive environment and demands from the team members skills beyond individual clinical skills. Thus, although teamwork should not be touted as a panacea for problems in interprofessional relations, it does create important opportunities for truly professional health care.

For Further Discussion

1. Discuss the doctor-nurse game. How have you seen it played? Is the nurse who plays it any less autonomous than one who refuses to play it? Explain. Is it a skill that all nurses should acquire?

2. We identified the fact that the nurse is usually an employee of the hospital as a significant factor when she finds herself in a conflict. Some hospitals are using the services of nursing pools to alleviate staffing problems. A nurse may work directly for a nursing pool but still work in the hospital. When she does so, she is not an employee of the hospital. Do you think this is a satisfactory alternative to working directly for a hospital? Does it create additional problems for the nurse who wishes to practice in a truly professional way? How might this type of relationship between the nurse and the hospital benefit or harm the quality of patient care? Research your answer by finding out how these pools are actually used in your community.

3. What kinds of experiences have you had during your nursing education that have helped prepare you to function as a member of an interprofessional health care team? What other experiences would be helpful in preparing you for this role?

4. Sections in this chapter have emphasized the relationship between nurses and physicians. What other professionals or groups do nurses interact with in their professional roles? How do relationships with these individuals or groups resemble or differ from nurses' relationships with physicians? What factors might contribute to those similarities and differences?

5. Many nursing leaders believe that all nurses should be taught assertiveness skills.

What is assertiveness? What is the relationship between assertive behavior and professional autonomy and accountability?

Bibliography

Aiken, L. H. (editor) (1982). Nursing in the 1980's: Crises, Opportunities, Challenges. Philadelphia: J. P. Lippincott Company.

Alfano, G. J. (1981). Joint Practice: A Collaborative Venture. In McClosky, J. C. and Grace, H.K., editors (1981). Current Issues in Nursing. Boston: Blackwell Scientific Publications, Inc.

American Medical Association (1983). Survey and Data Resources Excerpts. September, 1983.

American Nurses' Association (1985). Code for Nurses with Interpretive Statements. Kansas City, Missouri: The Association.

American Nurses' Association (1981). Inventory of Registered Nurses, 1977-78. Kansas City, Missouri: The Association.

American Nurses' Association (1981). Guidelines for Establishing Joint or Collaborative Practice in Hospitals. Kansas City, Missouri: The Association.

Annas, G. J. (1978). Informed Consent. Annual Review of Medicine, 29:9.

Ashley, J. A. (1976). Hospitals, Paternalism, and the Role of the Nurse. New York: Teachers' College Press.

Baker, K. (1980). Care of the Sick and Cure of Disease: Comment on the Fractured Image. In Spicker, S. and Gadow, S., editors (1980). Nursing: Images and Ideals. New York: Springer.

Bardwick, J. and Douvan, E. (1971). Ambivalence: The Socialization of Women. In Gornick, V. and Moran, B., editors (1971). Women in Sexist Society: Studies in Power and Powerlessness. New York: Basic Books.

Beauchamp, T. L. and Childress, J. F. (1979). Principles of Biomedical Ethics. New York: Oxford University Press.

Cassileth, B. R., Zupkis, R. V., Sutton-Smith, K. and March, V. (1980). Informed Consent: Why Are Its Goals Imperfectly Realized? New England Journal of Medicine, 302(16), April 17.

Cohen, H. (1981). The Nurse's Quest for a Professional Identity. California: Addison-Wesley Publishing Company.

Curtin, L. and Flaherty, M. J. (1982). Nursing Ethics: Theories and Pragmatics. Maryland: Robert J. Brady Company.

Davis, A. J. and Aroskar, M. A. (1983). Ethical Dilemmas and Nursing Practice. 2nd Edition. Norwalk, Connecticut: Appleton-Century-Crofts.

Ducanis, A. J. and Golin, A. K. (1979). The Interdisciplinary Health Care Team. Maryland: Aspen Systems.

Erde, E. L. (1982). Logical Confusions and Moral Dilemmas in Health Care Teams. In Agich, G. L., editor (1982). Responsibility in Health Care Teams. Boston: Reidell-Holland.

French, P. (ed.) (1972). Individual and Collective Responsibility. Cambridge, Massachusetts: Shenkman.

Gadow, S. (1980). Existential Advocacy: Philosophical Foundation of Nursing. In Spicker, S. and Gadow, S., editors (1980). Nursing: Images and Ideals. New York: Springer.

Gargaro, W. J. (1978a). Informed Consent. A Specific Case. Cancer Nursing, August, p. 329.

Gargaro, W. J. (1978b). Informed Consent. Update on the Tuma Case. Cancer Nursing, December, p. 467.

Holder, A. R. (1977). Legal Issues in Pediatric and Adolescent Medicine. New York: John Wiley and Sons.

Kalisch, B. J. (1975). Of Half Gods and Mortals: Aesculapian Authority. Nursing Outlook, 23(1):22.

Langham, P. (1979). Parental Consent: Its Justification and Limitations. Clinical Research, 27(5):301.

Lee, A. (1979a). Still the Handmaiden: How Nurses Rate with Physicians. RN, July, p. 21.

Lee, A. (1979b). We Want You, We Need You: How Nurses Rate with the Public. RN, June, p. 25.

Lever, J. (1976). Sex Differences in the Games Children Play. Social Problems, 23:478.

Lewis, E. P. (1977). The Right to Inform (Editorial). Nursing Outlook, 25:561.

Lewis, F. M. (1976). The Nurse as Lackey: A Sociological Perspective. Supervisor Nurse, April, p. 24.
Mappes, E. J. K. (1981). Ethical Dilemmas for Nurses: Physicians' Orders versus Patients' Rights. In Mappes, T. A. and Zembaty, J. S. (1981). Biomedical Ethics. New York: McGraw-Hill.
Mappes, T. A. and Zembaty, J. S. (1981). Biomedical Ethics. New York: McGraw-Hill.
Meleis, A. I. and Dagenais, F. (1981). Sex-Role Identity and Perception of Professional Self. Nursing Research, 30(3):162.
Muff, J. (1982). Joint Practice. In Muff, J., editor. Socialization, Sexism, and Stereotyping: Women's Issues in Nursing. St. Louis: C. V. Mosby Company.
Muhlenkamp, A. F. and Parsons, J. L. (1972). Characteristics of Nurses: An Overview of Recent Research Published in a Nursing Research Periodical. Journal of Vocational Behavior, 2:261.
Mussacchio, R. A. and Hough, D. E. , editors (1981). Socioeconomic Issues of Health—1981. Center for Health Policy Research: American Medical Association.
Mussen, P. H. (1969). Early Sex-role Development. In Goslin, D. A., editor (1969). Handbook of Socialization Theory and Research. Chicago: Rand-McNally.
Ozar, D. (1982). Three Models of Group Choice. The Journal of Medicine and Philosophy, 7:43.
Rein, I. (1977). Medical and Nursing Students: Concepts of Self and Ideal Self, Typical and Ideal Work Partner. Journal of Personality Assessment, 41(4):368.
Resser, D. and Shroder, A. K. (1980). Patient Interviewing: The Human Dimension. Baltimore: Williams and Wilkins.
Roth, L. H., Meisel, A., Lidz, C. W. (1977). Tests of Competency to Consent to Treatment. American Journal of Psychiatry, 134:3.
Russo, G. (1980). Are Nurses Getting Uppity? Journal of the Cincinnati Medical Society, Summer, p. 5.
Siegler, M. (1977). Critical Illness: The Limits of Autonomy. Hastings Center Report, 7:35.
Smith, M. D. (1982). The Virtuous Organization. Journal of Medicine and Philosophy, 7:35.
Smoyak, S. A. (1977). Problems in interprofessional relations. Bulletin of the New York Academy of Medicine, 53(Jan-Feb):51.
Sprunck, T. (1980). Sex-Role Identity and Image of Nursing. Nursing Research, 29(5):295.
Stanley, T. (1979). Is it Ethical to Give Hope to a Dying Person? Nursing Clinics of North America, 14:69.
Stanley, T. (1982). Ethical Reflections on the Tuma Case: Is It Part of the Nurse's Role to Advise on Alternate Forms of Therapy or Treatment? In McCloskey, J. C. and Grace, H. K., editors (1982). Current Issues in Nursing, Boston: Blackwell Scientific Publications, Inc.
Starr, P. (1982). The Social Transformation of American Medicine. New York: Basic Books.
Stein, L. I. (1967). The doctor-nurse game. Archives of General Psychiatry, 16:699.
Tait, K. M. and Winslow, G. (1977). Beyond Consent: The Ethics of Decision Making in Emergency Medicine. Western Journal of Medicine, 126(2):156.
Temkin-Greener, H. (1983). Interprofessional Perspectives on Teamwork in Health Care: A Case Study. Millbank Memorial Fund Quarterly, 61(4):641.
Till, T. S. (1980). Sex-Role Identity and Image of Nursing. Nursing Research, 29(5):295.

Chapter Seven

KNOWLEDGE AND THE EDUCATIONAL IMPERATIVE

Some of the most emotional and divisive controversies about nursing concern the kinds of knowledge nurses need and the institutions most appropriate for offering them that knowledge. This chapter will examine how knowledge and education relate to living and working as a professional nurse. It will look at nursing's educational system as it has developed and show how the history of nursing education has resulted in the controversies and unresolved issues it now faces. Then it will look at the problems faced by nurses in research, i.e., in the creation of new knowledge. Finally, it will offer some philosophical reflections on the nature of nursing knowledge in relation to other areas of knowledge.

KNOWLEDGE AND PROFESSIONALISM: INDIVIDUAL AND COLLECTIVE DUTY

Although ignorance may sometimes be bliss, sheer prudence dictates that it is better to know what you are doing than to operate in a fog. For members of the professions, being expert is more than a matter of personal pride; it becomes a matter of professional ethics. Clients come to a professional expecting and trusting that the professional has knowledge and expertise that the client needs but does not have. The implicit promise that the professional makes in accepting a client or patient involves their mutual understanding that the professional has a special knowledge and will use it for the benefit of the client. Thus, knowledge and expertise form an integral part of the individual professional's promise to each client and become an ethical duty for the individual member of the profession.

When a highly complex expertise is sought, clients' lack of knowledge prevents them from judging for themselves that the practitioner is competent. In regarding some occupations as professions, society is indicating that it expects the members of that occupational group to make sure that its practitioners have adequate knowledge. Clients assume, when dealing with the professions, that whoever bears a professional title (be it physician, nurse, or other title) has expert knowledge. Individual physicians, nurses, attorneys, and members of other professional groups are judged to be competent by the very fact that they are members of the profession. An occupational group that accepts for itself the designation "profession" makes society's expectation legitimate. Consequently, there is a collective ethical duty of the profession as a whole to ensure that relevant knowledge is available and that its members have and use that knowledge.

Professions themselves thus become responsible for certifying the competence of the graduates of their educational programs. The duty to maintain expertise is thus a collective one for the profession and cannot be met alone by the private actions of individual members. This collective responsibility is translated into action only when individual members of the profession take it upon themselves to maintain the good faith of their profession's promise to society. There are at least three dimensions to the ethical duty of the professional to maintain expertise: the duty that each professional owes each client, the collective duty that the profession owes society to ensure the expertise of each of its members, and the duty of individual professionals to discharge the collective duty of their profession. In what follows we will refer to this web of individual obligation and the collective obligation of the profession to maintain expertise as the *educational imperative*. There have been a variety of responses to the imperative, and they have led to controversies that are still not entirely resolved.

PROFESSIONAL AND TECHNICAL NURSING—A DIVIDED HOUSE?

Should basic nursing education emphasize a broad general education and theoretical knowledge? Or should beginning nursing programs place major emphasis on the acquisition of technical skills? Should "professional" nursing be distinguished from "technical" nursing? How much education is necessary for competent professional nursing practice? What is the best type of educational institution to provide appropriate education?

Nursing has struggled with these and similar questions about the nature and purpose of nursing education since before the turn of the century. Even in the 1980's, after nearly 100 years of controversy, debates about education are often heated and emotional. Ostensibly the debates focus on the need for a distinction between technical and professional education and the necessary educational requirements for each. But the debate occurs within a social context with a variety of participants whose interests differ. A brief survey of the elements of nursing history that led to the divisions in nursing education will be illuminating. Then we will look briefly at what those divisions mean for the profession of nursing in the 1980's.

The Development of Nursing Education

The first organized nursing education of modern times began in Kaiserswerth, Germany, in 1836 when a German pastor by the name of Fliedner established a training school for nursing deaconesses. In 1851 Florence Nightingale received her nursing training at Kaiserswerth. After serving in the Crimean War from 1854 to 1856, Nightingale established her famous Nightingale School at St.Thomas Hospital in London. Nightingale also wrote about nursing education, elaborating upon and adding to her own experience at Kaiserswerth. She believed that schools should correlate theory with practice and that nursing instructors should be paid for their work. She recommended that the director of a nursing program should be a nurse independent of the hospital board, and that the school of nursing should not be financially dependent on the hospital. The Kaiserswerth and Nightingale schools served as models for the first programs established in the United States.

The earliest attempts to formalize and upgrade nursing education in the United States were carried out by several diverse groups. The first nursing program in the United States was started at the New England Hospital for Women and Children in 1872 by Dr. Marie Zakrzewska. It was patterned after the Kaiserswerth School. One year later, three more nursing schools opened. Two of them, the Bellevue Training School for Nurses in New York City and the Connecticut Training School in New Haven, were started by philanthropic societies motivated by a concern for the improvement of patient care. They fashioned their programs after the Nightingale School in London. The Bellevue School was established despite resistance from local physicians, who did not believe formal training was necessary for nurses to perform their duties. They maintained that women who had received medical training would automatically consider themselves capable of practicing medicine and would immediately go out into the country and do so (Kalisch and Kalisch, 1986).

A third school, which opened the same year at the Massachusetts General Training School in Boston, was founded at the insistence of the Boston Women's Educational Union. This program was also modeled after the Nightingale School. One big difference was that housekeeping chores were removed from the student nurses' responsibilities and delegated to attendants. This group's conception of nursing as a career opportunity influenced what they believed to be necessary content in a nursing education program.

During the late nineteenth and early twentieth centuries a large number of nursing schools were started by hospital administrators. By conducting a school of nursing, they had a ready supply of student nurses to provide staffing for the hospital. These students worked in exchange for their room, board, and education. It was also common practice to send student nurses into patient homes to provide care. Home care patients reimbursed the hospital for the care provided by students. Thus the presence of students provided both indirect and direct sources of income for the hospital. Moreover, having a nurse training program on the premises ensured the hospital of a steady source of nurses who had completed the program. Hospital administrators who depended upon the students' contributions to the economic stability of the institution were not easily convinced that students needed large blocks of classroom experience that took them from the hospital wards.

These early efforts in nursing education were all efforts by groups other than nurses. Each of these groups viewed nursing roles from different perspectives. The physician wanted a technically skilled assistant; the hospital administrator valued a readily available student; the women's group wanted an attractive career choice for women. Since each group perceived nursing roles differently, each had somewhat different ideas about how nurses should be trained. Nurses themselves played a minor role in the early development of nursing education primarily because of their lack of training. At this point in its history, nursing was not expected by society to be a profession. Nurses were employees and technical assistants and their preparation was being determined by other groups.

But nurses recognized that they had a duty to improve the quality of nursing care being provided in hospitals at that time. They linked better care to better training for practitioners, and as early as 1876 nurses themselves were striving for better nursing education (Flanagan, 1976). Graduates of the first programs quickly became involved in a movement to standardize the quality of education across the country.

Isabelle Hampton Robb, one of the first graduates of the Bellevue Training School, was instrumental in 1893 in establishing the Society of Superintendents of Training Schools, the first formal professional organization in nursing and precursor to the National League for Nursing. She served also as the first president of the Nurses Associated Alumnae of the U.S. and Canada, the precursor of the American Nurses' Association. In such early efforts to organize, we can see the beginnings of collective efforts by nurses to ensure the educational competence of nurses.

These early organizations provided a basis for the state licensure movement, a significant development that directly affected nursing education. Robb and her colleagues recognized that there were wide variations in the quality of nursing education and resulting variations in the quality of practitioners. No regulatory mechanisms then existed and there were no uniform standards for educational programs. The bases and structures of programs varied with the motives of their diverse organizers. Consequently, individuals with little or no formal education often worked as nurses, and patients had no way of knowing how well qualified a given nurse was. Nursing was not yet in a position to offer consistent expertise, and society did not expect it to do so. Society and nursing were not yet ready to made nursing a profession.

In her reform efforts, Robb stressed the disservice and inequity to patients of this state of affairs in nursing education. She encouraged all nurses to work within their own states to establish *nurse practice acts*. These laws would establish minimum standards for training programs and minimum qualifications for those who practice nursing. The effort to establish state licensure laws was an undertaking of major proportions to a women's occupation during that era: women did not yet have the right to vote. By 1920, 47 of the 48 states had some type of nurse practice act. Today nurse practice acts continue to be the focal point of efforts to reform the nursing profession.

At the same time they were campaigning for state licensure, nurses were planning for the future of education. The Society of Superintendents recognized the increasing demand for well–trained nurses and a variety of new practice settings for nurses who had better qualifications. They worked to raise student entrance requirements and to establish nursing programs within the university setting. The first true baccalaureate degree program in nursing was established at Yale University in 1925.

The movement of nursing into the university setting was significant for three reasons. First, it was a major step in upgrading and standardizing nursing education. Nursing programs and their faculties had to meet standards similar to those of other university programs. Students entering nursing had to meet the same admission criteria as other students. By entering the university community, nursing demonstrated its readiness to meet the same rigorous standards applied to other academic programs—a major step in accepting the educational obligations of a profession.

Second, in entering the university, nurses were accepting a set of values about education that characterize the university. A university education is more than preparation for a career; it is preparation for the challenges of life itself. In the university the acquisition of technical skills is secondary to the acquisition of a broad general education that includes analytical thinking skills and an appreciation for lifelong learning. University students are taught by faculty who are specialists in a variety of disciplines. These faculty challenge the students to test a variety of perspectives from which the world and our experience of it can be understood. The presence of other students who are not in nursing has a similar broadening effect. Nursing students educated in the university setting develop a broader perspective on their practice and the social environment in which it occurs than do students whose training is exclusively devoted to technical skills.

A third reason why the move to the university was important is the primary emphasis on education to be found in the university. When education occurs within an institution whose primary role is education, the goal of administrative and academic decision-making is the educational experience. In contrast, an institution such as a hospital exists primarily for the purpose of providing services. Of necessity, administrative and financial decisions must be made with service as their goal. When service needs and training needs conflict service needs necessarily take priority.

Certainly the university's broad perspective is an advantage, but it should be remembered that such a broad perspective can create problems for professional education within academia. The university as a whole bears the responsibility for the quality of each of its programs and makes significant decisions concerning the content of those programs. But the professional curriculum must be determined by the skills and knowledge necessary for direct entry into the world of professional practice. Moreover, professional education must meet not only university standards but also the standards of professional accrediting groups (such as the National League for Nursing) and state requirements for licensure. In the university, professional programs must compete for available resources with other unrelated programs. In short, the broad perspective of a university creates a diversity of demands on professional programs. These demands may be appropriate, but they may also be inappropriate for the eventual goal of professional practice.

The early preparation of nurses for public health nursing provides a good example of what happens when educational goals become too narrowly focused on the current practice situation. After the founding of the American Public Health Association in 1872, activities in public health increased. In 1891, 130 nurses devoted all of their time to public health nursing (in activities such as home care, safety inspections, school health programs, alcohol control, and teaching about health, safety, and sanitation). By 1919 that number had increased to nearly 9000 (Brainard, 1922). Few nurses who entered public health received training other than their hospital training.

In 1920 that state of affairs culminated in the famous *Goldmark Report.* This study, undertaken initially through the intervention of Adelaide Nutting, a prominent nursing leader of the time, began to investigate the "proper training of the public health nurse" because of a recognition that nursing was not keeping pace with developments in the field of public health (American Journal of Nursing, April, 1920). Nursing's deficiencies in public health were due in some part to the fact that most nurses were trained in hospitals to work in hospital settings. The report noted that there was widespread neglect of public health nursing in existing nursing programs, that nursing programs varied widely in quality, that faculty were often poorly qualified, and that generally the individual in charge of nursing education was also in charge of nursing service. It recommended that nursing service and education be separated, that programs increase their emphasis on the relationship between theory and practice, and that stronger ties with the university be instituted (Goldmark, 1923). The establishment of the program at Yale, which contained a strong emphasis on public health nursing, was a first direct result of this study.

The movement of nursing education into universities could have become a strong visible sign of nursing's willingness to respond to the educational imperative implicit in professional commitment. That did not happen, because higher education for nurses met with a great deal of resistance from both outside and inside the ranks of nursing. Hospital administrators initially resisted for fear that hospitals could not afford to pay graduate nurses to replace student workers and later on the grounds that the hospital schools were uniquely capable of preparing a competent practitioner. Physicians resisted more sophisticated education for nurses because they valued nurses in their role as uneducated but devoted caregiver and feared that more educated nurses would attempt to practice medicine.

Nursing's status was undoubtedly affected by the status of women during the early part of the century. Nursing was one of the few acceptable career choices for women and was considered to a great extent a natural extension of mothering at a time when collegiate education for women was less accepted. Public opinion concerning education for women in general offered little support to nurses' efforts to improve their educational status.

Nursing training in hospital programs often resulted in strong loyalties to these programs. As we have already noted, hospital schools placed much emphasis on service to the institution. Students were taught to work long hours performing any and all duties associated with hospital care. They were taught to be grateful to the institution that provided them room, board, and a chance to become a graduate nurse. Many hospital schools were conducted under the auspices of hospitals run by religious orders of deaconesses or nuns. These religious groups also instilled in students a sense of dedication to service of the patients, often with a very direct religious dimension. The students of these programs often had strong loyalties to the hospitals that trained them, valued clinical practice, and sometimes feared that moving nursing programs away from hospitals would result in a loss of commitment.

The Current Controversy

Behind the disagreement about university-based education for nurses is an even more fundamental disagreement about the nature of nursing itself. Persons who favor collegiate education are for the most part those individuals who believe that nursing is an area of practice separate from and complementary to medicine. Nurses assist physicians, but they also perform independent nursing functions and are accountable directly to the patients they serve as their clients as well as to the physician. Because nurses perform independent functions and make decisions about patient care, they need a thorough understanding of the theory underlying practice and the ability to function in a variety of settings in and out of the hospital.

Persons who oppose collegiate education have often held a more traditional and conservative view of the nurse's role, maintaining that assisting the physician is still the primary nursing role and that proficiency in performing clinical technical activities is more important than theoretical knowledge.

Gradually these two views of nursing have become differentiated as *professional* and *technical* practice roles. The distinction was first made with the introduction of associate degree nursing programs in the 1950's. Associate degree education was introduced as an alternative to hospital-based education as a way of preparing a beginning level technical practitioner in two years while moving nursing education out of the hospital and into a general education setting. Baccalaureate-prepared nurses were to be considered beginning professional nurses and would be prepared to assume more diverse responsibilities and function in more complex roles.

The technical/professional distinction was formalized by the ANA in 1965 when it issued a position paper on education for nursing. In this paper the association endorsed the baccalaureate degree as minimum preparation for the practice of professional nursing and the associate degree as minimum preparation for technical nursing. Later, the association issued a stronger resolution calling for implementation of the baccalaureate requirement by 1985. The 1985 goal was not met, but in that year the ANA reaffirmed its stand and the National League for Nursing supported it.

These positions by the professional association have created tremendous controversy among nurses. The tension between the two differing views of nursing education that had existed since before the turn of the century culminated in heated debates over the "1985 proposal." Debate focused more on the survival of traditional hospital programs than on the real issue of what knowledge base was essential for truly professional nursing practice. Participants seemed to lose track of nurses' common commitment to providing the best possible care for their clients.

The question of appropriate educational institutions and appropriate education for nurses is still a hotly contested one. There are ethical questions that must be answered. First is the question of nursing's professional promise to society. In order to decide the appropriate nature, amount, and setting of nursing education one must first clarify the nature of the profession's promise or contract with society. That promise includes not only what nurses want to offer to society but also what society expects of them. The education of nurses must be consistent with the basic contract between nursing and society. Nurses may legitimately attempt to convince the public that more can be expected of nursing than society currently wants. Success in raising society's demands on the nursing profession would bring with it the imperative of an education consistent with those new demands. But nursing's professional status and the ethical duties of that status remain a function of the voluntary arrangement between society and nursing.

Second, there are utilitarian considerations involved in determining the amount of education necessary. The cost of the various forms of education and their effect on the cost of health care must be weighed against the potential benefit to society of having nurses educated at that level. Alternative available educational requirements must be explored. In addition, the effect of educational requirements on the number of persons entering nursing may well have some effect on the quality of health care delivered.

Perhaps the controversy over education has been necessary to the evolution of nursing as a profession. If so, evolution into professionalism cannot continue until nurses come to grips with this important issue. The relationship between a profession and society is based on the mutual understanding of what members of the profession have promised to do for their clients. Implicit in the relationship is the trust that the profession will decide what knowledge is necessary to perform professional services and will ensure that all practitioners have that knowledge. The issue facing nurses now is when and how nursing will meet this step toward professionalism. Continued division makes it difficult for a patient to know what to expect. It is an indication that this basic problem of professional life confounds nursing, even if individual practitioners are competent and sincere.

NURSING RESEARCH

The educational process involves more than the transmission of nursing knowledge from those who already have it to those who aspire to it. Also, professional nursing practice involves more than simply applying an unchanging body of knowledge. Knowledge in general is not static; it develops and grows. In order to ensure that practitioners are providing the best possible care, members of the profession must continually seek to improve that care in the light of new knowledge. Through nursing research, nurses expand the profession's knowledge base and discover ways to apply that knowledge in clinical practice for the benefit of their patients.

Nurses are now taught to appreciate the interrelationship of research, practice, and education. Researchers frequently address questions raised by educators and practitioners. They relay their findings to practitioners, who incorporate them into practice, thus continually applying the latest knowledge for the benefit of the client. Educators likewise incorporate the researcher's findings into their educational programs, thus ensuring that new nurses entering the profession have the most relevant and up-to-date knowledge possible. The ongoing exchange among these three centers of professional activity provides the foundation for the continual development of the profession's body of knowledge.

Because this exchange is essential to fulfillment of the educational imperative, all members of the profession ought to contribute to the research-practice-education dialogue in some way. A few assume the role of full-time researcher. Others become educators. Most of the members of the profession function as practitioners; they support the development of knowledge by raising questions in their everyday practice and by incorporating research findings into their practice. After looking at how nursing research has developed in this century, we will examine more carefully some of the ethical questions posed by the acquisition of new knowledge, questions for the nurse-researcher as well as for the nurse who is more involved in practice than in research.

Nursing research is not simply research done by people who happen to be nurses. It is a vital component of the educational imperative and is essential to the continued offering of quality care.

> Nursing research develops knowledge about health over the full lifespan, care of persons with health problems and disabilities, and nursing actions to enhance the ability of individuals to respond effectively to actual or potential health problems. . . . Research conducted by nurses includes various types of studies in order to derive clinical interventions to assist those who require nursing care (American Nurses' Association, 1981).

The Development of Nursing Research

Florence Nightingale is often considered the founder of modern nursing education. She was also the first nursing researcher. Nightingale kept detailed records of her observations about the effects of nursing care in the Crimea as well as detailed epidemiological statistics that were used to improve the English military hospital system. Except for Nightingale's early efforts, however, the nurse as a researcher is a relatively recent phenomenon. During the first half of the twentieth century professional efforts were focused on improving the skills of the practitioner and the nurse educator, on the basis of knowledge already available. Little emphasis was placed on augmenting the knowledge base or seeking evidence for the effectiveness of nursing interventions. Gradually, particularly in the 1950's, research became recognized as an integral part of professional nursing life.

The establishment of the Institute of Research and Service in Nursing Education at Columbia University in 1953 was a major early milestone in the development of nursing research. This was the first formalized mechanism within a university to carry out nursing research. The institute was established to conduct research on selected problems in nursing and nursing education, to disseminate the results of research undertaken by the institute, and to assist in the preparation of nurses for the conduct of research in nursing (Abdellah and Levine, 1979).

The American Nurses' Association has played a vital role in the development of nursing research in the U.S. In 1952 it began publication of *Nursing Research*, the organization's first official journal for reporting research related to nursing and health. In 1955 the ANA established the American Nurses' Foundation, which was devoted solely to the promotion of nursing research through financial support and the dissemination of research findings. The professional association has also nurtured research activities through its Commission on Nursing Research, established in 1970 to formulate policy concerning research, to recommend priorities for the profession's research concerns, and to participate in the establishment of standards of nursing research (Flanagan, 1976). It was this body that prepared documents such as *Human Rights Guidelines for Nurses in Clinical and Other Research* (1974) and *Priorities for Nursing Research* (1976).

The *Priorities for Nursing Research* pointed out the reality that clinical nursing research was being neglected in favor of other kinds of projects. As the document explains, the development of research priorities would

> . . . assist the profession to focus on and direct its action toward developing the knowledge and information that is needed as a basis for improving the practice of nursing and advancing the profession.

The Commission re-emphasized the need for clinical research in 1981:

> Accountability to the public for the humane use of knowledge in providing effective and high quality services is the hallmark of a profession. Thus, the preeminent goal of scientific inquiry by nurses is the ongoing development of knowledge for use in the practice of nursing (American Nurses' Association, 1981).

During the 1970's the number of published studies dealing with clinical issues began to increase. Both the ANA and the National League for Nursing began to emphasize the need for all students, graduate and undergraduate, to be prepared to interpret and even to engage in research. Graduate and undergraduate curricula now contain content on the research process. Some undergraduate curricula require students to carry out a carefully constructed research project of their own. Earned doctorates (which ordinarily require a substantial original research effort) have substantially increased. Regional and national meetings for the presentation of research findings as well as several new research-oriented journals have appeared. In 1985 the National Center for Nursing Research in the National Institutes of Health was established.

The increasing awareness among nurses that they have direct obligations to their clients has brought with it the recognition that involvement in research is an ethical imperative, an important corollary to the *educational imperative*. The 1985 revision of the Code for Nurses summarizes this well in stating that

> Ongoing scholarly activity such as research and the development of theory is indispensable to the full discharge of a profession's obligations to society. Each nurse has a role in this area of professional activity . . . (Code for Nurses, 7.1).

The Ethics of Nursing Research: Consent and Autonomy

Active involvement in nursing research satisfies one of nursing's ethical obligations. But involvement in research raises new ethical questions, especially when the research involves human subjects. The more persistent ethical problems in research occur because of the duty to respect and preserve the autonomy of the subject. We have already discussed in some detail the problems of ensuring the autonomy of patients. In a research situation, these problems become even more complicated than they are in a therapeutic intervention, for the intervention is not solely for the patient's own benefit. In fact, the patient becomes a means to further knowledge sought primarily for the purpose of aiding *other* persons in the future. The research subject often loses privacy, is inconvenienced, and in some cases is deprived of usual care or exposed to increased personal risk. If respect for autonomy demands the full consent of patients even when health care providers are acting for their benefit, that consent becomes doubly important when patients are used or inconvenienced for the benefit of others.

As Kant pointed out, using persons *merely* as means is unethical because it fails to respect persons as having their own goals and intentions (see Chapter 2). This is true even when the goal we hope to accomplish is a good one. Scrupulous attention to the consent process will ensure that patients are active and willing partners in the research and will thus restore their autonomy: they will be used as a means but it will be by their own consent.

An ethical consent process requires more than the proper signature on the proper form. It requires also that patients be properly informed about the nature of the experiment, about any possible risks that it might pose for them, and about anything else that reasonable persons might want to consider before making up their minds about whether to serve as subjects. This "reasonable person" criterion is not quite the same thing as what the researcher would want to know if placed in the same situation. Reasonable people differ among themselves about what they would take into account in making such a decision, so the goal of the researcher should be to provide all the information that might be considered relevant by even unusual individuals. An informed consent will always include

> an explanation of the study, the procedures to be followed, and their purposes; a description of physical risk or discomfort, any invasion of

privacy, and any threat to dignity; and the methods used to protect anonymity and to insure confidentiality. The subject needs also to receive a description of any benefits to the subject and/or to the development of new knowledge that potentially might be expected (American Nurses' Association, 1975).

These guidelines were not developed originally and exclusively for nurses. The document from which they were taken distills and applies to the nursing context the ethical insights of several important documents–the Nuremberg Code and the Declaration of Helsinki, which has been endorsed by the American Medical Association in its principles of medical ethics.

The excuse that a research subject "wouldn't understand" or might be "overly frightened" by information is not a valid reason for withholding it. If patients would withdraw from the experiment if they had complete information, then respect for their autonomy would require giving them the information to make that choice. Subjects in research are being asked to do something for the benefit of others. To do anything that will prevent them from freely deciding whether to participate is treating them merely as tools for our purposes rather than as persons.

Research performed by health care professionals who are ordinarily entrusted with the care of patients creates more complex problems in preserving autonomy of patients and research subjects. In professional-client relationships clients have the legitimate expectation (the *right*) that professionals will use their skills and services for the benefit of the client. Thus, patients assume that any inconvenience, pain, or risk that they undergo is necessary for the benefits they expect to get. This is an important element of consent for a therapeutic procedure. But when persons become subjects of an experiment, they must recognize that the primary goal of the researcher is the acquisition of new knowledge rather than the benefit of the subjects. Patients might not choose to undergo the procedure if its benefits will not go to them personally. Respect for autonomy requires respect for such a choice.

When the researcher occupies a second role as caregiver, it may be difficult for patients to know whether the risks they undergo are for their own benefit. Nurses who seek the consent of a research subject are in a difficult position to which they must be extremely sensitive. Patients are simply not accustomed to seeing nurses in research roles and are likely to confuse the nurse-researcher with a nurse in the more usual and familiar therapeutic role. It then becomes easy for the subject to make the implicit assumption that the nurse's request for consent amounts to a professional therapeutic recommendation even if the nurse states clearly the nontherapeutic intent of the research. Patients may consent to research, assuming falsely that it is for their own benefit. The difficulty might not be in any misinformation that the nurse-researcher had given the patient, but in the traditional image of the nurse that is more enduring than the efforts of any one nurse to amend it.

One nurse thus described her first field research experience (in which she observed an antepartal education class):

> Almost at once, I realized that, despite my frequent explanations of my research goals, the expectant parents I was observing had difficulty understanding what a nurse was doing conducting research. At first, the majority of the parents cast me in the more familiar nurse role—asking my opinion of the various aspects of prenatal care given in that institution, asking technical questions about the material covered in class, and, in one case, asking me to accompany them during their labor and delivery as a support person (May, 1980).

Reflecting on her experience, the same nurse asks the following important questions concerning informed consent:

> If subjects frequently misperceive the nurse-researcher role, then to whom has the research subject given consent—the nurse or the researcher? If the subject defines the situation as one in which he will interact with a nurse, is it possible that his expectations and decision-making processes in giving consent may differ from those in which he expects to interact with a researcher?

Although nursing research is becoming more common and is gradually being accepted as a necessary activity for professional nurses, this has become true only in the very recent past. For many years the sole emphasis of nursing was direct patient care. Nurses in the research role necessarily have a different priority in their interaction with the patient-subject. The ethical researcher never completely loses sight of the patient's well-being. But the research process may involve inconvenience or risk to the subject that would be avoided in the professional-client relationship. Such inconveniences are permissible only when the patient has knowingly consented to them. Once the patient has consented, nurse-researchers must be able to separate themselves from the more familiar therapeutic role and assume the objective role of the researcher.

The nurse involved in research in a clinical setting faces another possible problem with informed consent. Patients may easily fear that their consent to participate in a research project will determine whether they receive adequate care for their own problems. The fear is understandable when the institution caring for the patients and the institution sponsoring the research are one and the same and when the same professionals are providing care and conducting research as well. It is obviously unethical to make quality health care contingent upon willingness to serve as a research subject; that would amount to a form of coercion, and consent could no longer be freely given or withheld. Professionals in practice situations ought to make sure that their patients realize that willingness to serve as a research subject is not a condition for a professional-client relationship.

Research subjects retain all the same rights to freedom, information, and privacy that clients in a treatment situation do. The research situation is more complex, because the research in which they serve as subjects has an important goal that is not always the same as what is best for individual patients. For this reason, some authors have argued that young children or severely retarded persons should never be used for experimentation. They always require proxy consent, and no one should be allowed to give a proxy consent except for the benefit of the person (Ramsey, 1976).

If it is an ethical imperative to be engaged in research, it must also be ethically important to do it well. The same reasons that make research important make it important also that research be executed carefully and that all the demands of scientific method and careful research protocol be scrupulously observed. Moreover, when human research subjects are used, they often give their consent with the belief that their participation will provide some benefit to humankind. It is unlikely that they would give their consent to a procedure that inconveniences them or puts them at risk if they thought that the research would be invalidated by the poorly built protocol of the researcher. This constitutes a second ethical reason for doing research carefully: researchers owe a direct debt of careful work to the persons whom they use in their research.

In the face of ever more complex research situations, how can the well-meaning researcher make sure that the rights of subjects are not violated? All institutions that receive federal funds are now required to have *institutional review boards* (IRB) to examine research proposals both for adequate protocol and the protection of the rights of human subjects. Some researchers regard the IRB as an adversary, as an impediment to their research. In fact, a committee of one's peers can be quite helpful in ensuring that research is designed well and respects the human dignity of the persons it uses. The IRB can be a useful adjunct to our well-intentioned efforts. Qualified nurses, whether personally engaged in research or not, should assume that there is a professional responsibility to serve on such boards. It is a part of the duty of the various professions engaged in research to ensure that the board functions to serve its ethical purpose.

Nurse-researchers have a variety of written resources to which they can turn to gain a better understanding of the issues involved in research. A variety of philosophical literature sources exist that examine the ethics of research. Various professional associations have built similar lists of guidelines for research on the basis of these underlying philosophical principles. The American Nurses' Association has produced a statement, *Human Rights Guidelines for Nurses in Clinical and Other Research*, which is consistent with sound thinking about research ethics and can serve as a useful basic guide. Maintaining an ethical approach to research requires researchers to become familiar with basic ethical problems frequently encountered and to reflect on the ways in which their own projects deal with matters of ethical importance. Although involvement in research is a function of professional commitment, concern for the ethics of research stems from respect for humanity. This respect is owed by all to all, even when there is no profession involved.

Research and the Practitioner

In fact, nurses engaged in practice may not find themselves directly exposed to research situations. However, research is still a necessary response to the *educational imperative*, even for the professional nurse not involved directly in research. The imperative demands of all professionals that they develop and nurture in themselves a set of habits and attitudes that could best be summarized as an *open and inquiring mind*.

An inquiring mind is a professional virtue. The inquiring mind does more than follow some set of ethical rules. Certainly, ethics does include the rules that deserve priority in our lives, but it includes also our beliefs about what kinds of personal habits and qualities are *good* for a human being to develop so that they constitute a sort of second nature. Such qualities constitute *what we are* in addition to determining *what we do*. Qualities or habits considered good and worth developing as a form of self-improvement are called *virtues*.

Professional commitment does indeed bind the professional to some specific ethical rules that do not hold for everyone. (Not everyone in the world, for example, should feel obliged to follow the specifics about confidentiality that the Code for Nurses requires.) A professional who takes seriously the rules of professional ethics develops the personal qualities necessary to honor consistently the professional commitment, qualities that we call *professional virtues*.

The *inquiring mind* is one such virtue. The inquiring mind recognizes that all scientific knowledge is tentative and provisional. This is not the same thing as being skeptical. Skepticism involves suspending belief in the truth of everything because nothing is certain. In the long run, it results in not using any information because it might all turn out to be false. On the other hand, accepting our knowledge as tentative involves recognizing that it is the closest to the truth we have been able to come so far. Thus, the inquiring mind is ready to use knowledge, while remaining aware that what we now take for the truth may have to be revised should new facts present themselves.

This fundamental recognition of the tentativeness of knowledge has been the subject of extensive discussion by scientists and philosophers (Kuhn, 1970; Popper, 1959). Knowledge that is empirically based is always an attempt to make some sense of what we have already observed. If something new is observed or if some new explanation makes more sense out of what we have already observed, then we may have to revise what we thought we knew. The history of science in general, of medicine, and of nursing have all been subject to this process and will continue to be so. The inquiring mind will not be taken entirely by surprise if the nursing knowledge gained during initial training eventually becomes outdated. But the inquiring mind is not just passively expectant that the knowledge base will change. The professional with an inquiring mind uses available knowledge while alert to the necessity of revising it as new facts are discovered.

The nurse in practice need not (and should not) assume that only the researcher can be possessed of an inquiring mind. The practicing nurse who is attentive to the facts of practice becomes an active participant in the flow of knowledge. Being aware that new knowledge may lead to a "better way" of doing routine things is the hallmark of an inquiring mind. The inquiring mind has an alertness that constantly makes comparisons of practice situations to see what works best and is open to the many opportunities for new knowledge. These opportunities may come from co-workers (a new nurse with different training, a nurse with years of experience), other health care professionals, continuing education programs, and readings. They can come from a wide variety of sources, and not just from within the nursing profession. The inquiring mind is open to the insights of experts in other fields and ready to transform those insights into something that can be used in nursing practice.

The inquiring mind is more than the impetus to a set of actions; it is a mentality to be developed, something that must eventually become automatic and natural. It is a *virtue* because society has a right to expect that members of the professions that serve it have made a habit of inquiry, that they seek knowledge naturally and freely. To approach new knowledge with anything less than an inquiring mind is to fail the society for which the professions exist.

THE NATURE OF NURSING KNOWLEDGE AND A CONCLUSION

Though most professional nurses today would agree to the need for a scientific basis for practice, many disagree on what the nature of the scientific knowledge base should be. Two schools of thought have developed on this issue, and it may be helpful to briefly review both of them. One holds that there is a unique nursing science that is distinct from but just as basic and legitimate as other sciences such as psychology, sociology, and biology. As a distinct science, nursing must have a body of knowledge that is unique to it and that will develop through "pure" nursing research, rather than by borrowing knowledge from other basic sciences.

The second viewpoint is that nursing has as its knowledge base an applied science. An applied science, rather than having a separate, distinct body of knowledge, applies knowledge from other sciences to its area of concern. Proponents of nursing as an applied science point out that nursing applies knowledge of physiology, chemistry, psychology, sociology, and other sciences to specific nursing practice situations. In this view, the concepts and basic information that form the fundamental building blocks from which nursing knowledge is created are not unique to nursing. In nursing, just as in medicine and other practical disciplines, these fundamental concepts and methods are reorganized in a way that describes nursing activities and explains and predicts their outcomes (Walker, 1971). A professional discipline transforms basic, shared knowledge according to the unique goals of that profession. It is in this sense that it seems most reasonable to say that nursing (or any other profession) has a unique knowledge base: the nature of nursing practice transforms shared knowledge into something unique to nursing.

It is possible to mentally separate the activity of nursing from the expert knowledge that professional nurses use. Nursing would not have to be a profession; however, if it is, it must undertake to establish a connection between these two separate entities, the knowledge base and the activity of nursing. A profession takes it upon itself to ensure that the activity does not occur without an adequate knowledge base. In summary, that is what we mean when we claim that the professions have an *educational imperative*. Nursing as a profession is a scientific art, and establishing and preserving the connection between science and practice are part of what the professional has promised to do.

For Further Discussion

1. "Grandfathering" is a legislative provision that makes new legislation inapplicable to a previously existing circumstance. For example, if a state introduces the professional-technical nurse distinction into its nurse practice act, it might declare that all nurses previously licensed will be treated as professional nurses and will have all their rights and duties. Discuss the pros and cons of such a move by a state legislature. What general principles would you use to explain your support or lack of support for grandfathering?

2. All institutions who receive government support and conduct research must now have institutional review boards (IRB) which must first approve research projects that use human subjects. Choose a hospital or other institution with which you are familiar and examine the procedure that is used to get the approval of the IRB. Explain how that procedure is intended to protect the rights and welfare of the research subject.

3. Consider the following situation:

   You direct the nursing service in a long-term care facility. One of your major vendors meets with you to discuss introducing a new bed pad for your patients. The pads you now use are effective. The company wants to test a new one to see if it causes allergic or other adverse reactions. The company will provide the pads to you at low cost and also make a small donation to support your day activities program for the next six

months if you will do a two-month trial of the pads on one half of the incontinent patients in your unit. (The activities program is in danger of being severely cut back because of a lack of funds.) The company has heard anecdotal reports that some of its pads have caused mild irritation to sensitive individuals. Its own extensive tests do not confirm those reports. The vendor is hoping that you will help him show the rest of the market that there is no problem with the pads.

Explain how this is similar and dissimilar to human research. Put together a list of the questions you would want to resolve with the supplier before making your decision. Then explain how these questions relate to the principles on which you would base a decision.

Bibliography

Abdellah, F. and Levine, E. (1979). Better Patient Care Through Nursing Research. New York: Macmillan Company.

American Nurses' Association (1966). American Nurses' Association First Position on Education for Nursing. American Journal of Nursing, 66:515.

American Nurses' Association (1975). Human Rights Guidelines for Nurses in Clinical and Other Research. Kansas City, Missouri: The Association.

American Nurses' Association (1976). Priorities for Nursing Research. Kansas City, Missouri: The Association.

American Nurses' Association (1981). Research Priorities for the 1980's. Kansas City, Missouri: The Association.

American Nurses' Association (1985). Code for Nurses with Interpretive Statements. Kansas City, Missouri: The Association.

Brainard, A. M. (1922). The Evolution of Public Health Nursing. Philadelphia, W. B. Saunders Company.

Davis, A. and Krueger, J. C. (1980). Patients, Nurses, Ethics. New York: American Journal of Nursing Company.

Flanagan, L. (1976). One Strong Voice: The Story of the American Nurses' Association. Kansas City, Missouri: American Nurses' Association.

Freund, P. (editor) (1970). Experimentation with Human Subjects. New York: George Braziller.

Goldmark, J. C. (1923). Nursing and Nursing Education in the United States. New York: Macmillan Company.

Kalisch, P. A. and Kalisch, B. J. (1986). The Advance of American Nursing. 2nd Edition. Boston: Little, Brown and Company.

Kuhn, T. S. (1970). The Structure of Scientific Revolutions. 2nd Edition. Chicago: University of Chicago Press.

May, K. A. (1980). Informed Consent and Role Conflict. In Davis, A. and Krueger, J. C. editors (1980). Patients, Nurses, Ethics. New York: American Journal of Nursing Company.

Montag, M. L. (1963). Technical Education in Nursing. American Journal of Nursing, 63:100.

Parsons, T. (1970). Research with Human Subjects and the "Professional Complex." In Freund, P., editor (1970). Experimentation with Human Subjects. New York: George Braziller.

Popper, K. (1959). The Logic of Scientific Discovery. New York: Harper and Row.

Ramsey, P. (1976). The Enforcement of Morals: Nontherapeutic Research on Children. Hastings Center Reports, 6:41.

Walker, L. O. (1971). Toward a Clearer Understanding of the Concept of Nursing Theory. Nursing Research, 20(5):428.

Chapter Eight

THE ECONOMIC SITUATION IN NURSING

At first thought, a discussion of economics may seem out of place in a book about professional ethics. The relevance of issues such as the demand for nursing services or third-party reimbursement to ethical practice may not seem readily apparent. Yet the number and quality of nurses available to provide patient care are controlled to a great degree by the economic market in which nurses practice. Thus, economic issues have important implications for the practice of truly professional nursing.

Nurses, like members of all other occupational groups, want to be adequately compensated for the services they provide. In most occupations this is not controversial: it is generally expected that workers will seek the highest possible wage for their work. In nursing, however, the traditional culture has regarded self-interest in the pursuit of wages as opposed to nurses' commitment to patient care.

Although nursing leaders have often emphasized the importance of the economic status of the profession, nurses have for the most part been uncomfortable with pursuing their own interests in the marketplace. This discomfort is related to several social factors. One is the historical roots of nursing education in religiously affiliated institutions. The religious orders that controlled these institutions saw selfless devotion to others, poverty, and a simple life as the ideal; these values were embodied in their educational programs. Members of the religious communities who taught in such institutions had themselves taken lifelong vows of obedience and demonstrated great selflessness and loyalty to their institutions. It seemed quite natural that their students should do so as well. Nurses who felt an obligation to their patients and a sense of loyalty to their employers endured long working hours, performed menial tasks "for the good of the patient," and accepted the meager wages that were offered.

But the religious affiliation of much nursing education does not entirely explain nurses' reluctance to move for improved personal compensation. Like other female occupations, nursing was not valued as an occupation on a par with male occupations. Nursing roles have been perceived as a "natural" extension of mothering, something that was easy and natural for women because of their gender. Caring for and nurturing others was what women were supposed to do, not something for which they should expect compensation in the same way that skilled labor would be compensated. Both men and women held this attitude, and the stereotype did not begin to change until the 1960's and 1970's.

However, women are now essential to the economy; they do not come in and out of the workplace at will or remain in it just until they have children. We saw in Chapter 5 that more nurses are remaining fairly continuously employed in their adult years. This is due often to the necessity of a two-income family. But it is due also to the fact that women are now much more often the sole source of support of their families. In other words, the wages that women earn are no longer incidental. Thus women are concerned about adequate compensation for their services, because it is important to their own personal welfare and the welfare of those for whom women are primarily responsible.

It is a commonly held belief that people have the right to protect their own welfare. Claims to the right to basic health care and self-defense are applications of this belief. It is possible to reject this right, but in doing so one would have to reject many other rights that persons are generally believed to have. Thus there is some reason to believe that women, and members of predominantly female occupational groups such as nursing, are justified in their efforts to obtain adequate compensation. It follows that utter selflessness on the part of nurses then could be simply a refusal or inability to exercise a moral right.

The controversial ethical questions concern not the existence of such a right but the extent to which it can be acted upon, especially in situations in which that action begins to conflict with rights of other persons. In the health professions, the moral right to pursue personal welfare may conflict with the moral duty that professionals have to their patients. One approach to resolving such a conflict is to assume that the right to personal welfare always should take absolute priority and conclude that any assumed rights that clients have must always defer to nurses' rights to increased income, better hours, or some other personal benefit. Such an extreme position conflicts very directly with the professional commitment. Members of the professions have dependent clients and should not take advantage of their trust. When they do so, they violate professional ethics.

A more moderate position might be to try to find a "happy medium" between one's right to personal welfare and the rights that others have as a result of the person's proclaimed professional commitment. The attempt to strike such a balance leads to dilemmas in having to choose between one's own welfare and that of others. Making this kind of choice is difficult in all aspects of life, but it is particularly complex in professional-client situations. Professionals who seek to improve their economic situation must consider not only the rights of patients for whom they are currently caring but also the rights and needs of future patients. Likewise, they must also consider the impact of their actions on the profession as a whole and its relationship with society. To do this requires understanding of a number of other factors that complicate efforts to balance the nurse's personal welfare with the demands of professionalism.

THE CURRENT ECONOMIC STATUS OF NURSES

In 1984, according to statistics from the American Nurses' Association, the average starting salary for a staff or general duty registered nurse ranged from $18,768 to $25,272. Since nearly 70 per cent of all employed nurses are in hospitals working in general duty positions, these figures represent the salary range for the greatest majority of registered nurses. The figures are comparable to those for other predominantly female occupational groups such as teachers, who averaged $22,900 during 1984 and secretaries, whose average wages for the same year were $17,784. In contrast, during 1984 postal employees made $31,562, city sanitation workers averaged $29,892, public transit workers $27,672, and telephone employees $28,600.

There are also indications that nurses' wages have not kept pace with those of other health providers. In 1960, licensed practical nurse incomes were 70 per cent of registered nurse incomes. By 1980 practical nurses were making 76 per cent of what registered nurses were making. In contrast, the gap between the incomes of nurses and physicians has widened. In 1945, nurses incomes were one third of physicians' incomes; in 1983 nurses were making approximately one fifth of what physicians were making annually (Aiken, 1982; Dept. of Commerce, 1986).

Such figures are disturbing, but it is difficult to know what meaning to attach to them. One attempt to interpret wage differences between occupational groups as an issue of social justice is the concept of *comparable worth*. Comparable worth has been used in some situations to explain low salaries in nursing and justify demands for improvements (Rothman and Rothman, 1980). Another way to try to explain the status of nurses' wages is through the analysis of the market for nurses within the framework of an economic model of supply and demand. We will look at both of these approaches, noting the strengths and problems associated with each, and discuss the significance of economic issues to professional ethics.

COMPARABLE WORTH

In recent years, women working in predominantly male occupations who believed that they were underpaid have had legal recourse: the legal doctrine of equal pay for equal worth ensures that a woman who does the same work as a man must be paid at the same wage. But equal worth does nothing for those women who are clustered in occupations in which most of the workers are women. In such cases, it is possible for the whole occupation to be receiving a depressed wage, even though members within the occupational group are being treated equally. In the past it was difficult to demonstrate the inequity in women's wages in these situations, since it was impossible to point to a reference group that was receiving the "fair" wage and show how women's wage did not match it.

The criterion of equal pay for comparable worth proposes that different but comparable occupations be paid at the same rate. Two different occupations are said to be comparable when they are equal in terms of such factors as education required, complexity of skills, working conditions, and accountability (Brett, 1983). When comparable worth has been seriously applied, very detailed methods have been developed to enable diverse occupations to be compared to one another. The goal of such comparisons is to arrive at a common measure (often a point value) by which to decide if two different occupations are really comparable. If they are, then we might conclude that they ought to be compensated equally.

To draw such a conclusion is to claim that the marketplace should not be counted on to establish wages, and consequently that it should not be counted on to ensure that the necessary supply of labor is available. At the same time we would be presuming that we knew such things as the net benefit that the occupation provided. There are a number of weaknesses in both the theory and the application of comparable worth, not the least of which concerns with what other employment groups nursing should be considered comparable (Bunzel, 1981; Livernash, 1980; Remick, 1980).

Nurses in a number of states have used the criterion of comparable worth in pressing their demands for wage increases (Brett, 1983; AJN, 1983; McCarty, 1985). So far, the results in courtrooms where comparable worth suits have been considered have been mixed (see *Lemon v. City of Denver*; *Brennan v. Owensboro-Davies City Hospital*). Some groups and institutions, such as the U.S. Civil Rights Commission, oppose the use of comparable worth as a basis for ending pay discrimination against women. This group believes that the major reasons for wage differences between job categories is related to socialization factors rather than sex-based biases (McCarty, 1985). Comparable worth may eventually prove to be a useful tool to ensure equity of pay for nurses. But before it can become such, there are a number of difficult questions to be answered concerning its application. One, as noted, is the question of to what other groups nursing should be compared. Another is the issue of the actual value of nursing services.

The Worth of Nursing

One way of measuring the value of employees is by the wage required to get them to work—in other words, by the marketplace. However, there are other ways of measuring the value of an employee that are not a function of the minimum amount of money required to get that employee to work. We might, for example, measure an employee's worth by what that employee contributes through his or her labor. This element of contribution forms part of the framework of comparable worth. To attach a numerical value to a worker's contribution is difficult and controversial for any kind of labor. In the case of nursing, we can find some specific difficulties.

These difficulties are attributable, at least in part, to the fact that the nursing profession has failed to show clearly what nursing's contribution to patient care is. Even recent definitions of nursing fall short of providing quantifiable characteristics that can be used to establish how much of what kinds of skills are needed to meet the patient's needs.

Serious attempts are being made by nurses to address this important issue. One early attempt at devising a system of identifying and quantifying nursing services has been the *relative intensity measures* (RIM) system. RIM attempts to measure in minutes the intensity of nursing care required by patients in different diagnostic groupings (DRG's)(Grimaldi and Micheletti, 1982). This approach provides a mechanism for identifying and quantifying what nursing care is and what hospitals and patients are getting for their money.

There are a number of problems with the RIM system. One possible drawback is that it is designed to complement the medical diagnostic groupings. This necessarily emphasizes the medical model approach to nursing care that many nurses see as restrictive if not totally inappropriate. Although the decision to offer some aspects of nursing care is dependent on medical diagnosis, much of what nurses do is not strictly determined by the classifications used in medicine.

Preliminary work with the RIM system revealed that the system is fairly complex and cumbersome. Some evaluations have shown that applying the RIM formulas could artificially and inaccurately reduce the amount of reimbursement hospitals would receive for nursing care (Trofino, 1985). Other approaches to determining the cost of nursing care have relied upon already existing patient classification systems (Mitchell, et al, 1984; Prescott, 1986). The use of any of these measures presumes that we have already settled the question of what nursing consists of and are able to distinguish nursing from non-nursing work. As we have noted before, this is not necessarily the case.

A related attempt to clarify nursing practice is the development of a taxonomy of nursing diagnoses. Since 1973, the North American Nursing Diagnosis Association has conducted a major effort to define and standardize diagnoses made in the course of nursing care. This group sees the standardization of nomenclature and the classification of nursing diagnoses as an essential first step in facilitating communication about nursing's focus of concern and area of practice (Kim, McFarland and McLane, 1984). Once nursing diagnoses have been standardized, a system similar to the medical DRG's could be developed.

The RIM system, patient classification systems, and taxonomy of nursing diagnoses are approaches to specifying the contribution of nursing to patient care and establishing the value of the nurses' services to the institutions that employ them. The adequacy of such systems will be known only when the effect of nursing interventions on patient outcomes has been shown, and this will require systematic nursing research. These efforts may be stimulated by new reimbursement policies that will force employers to look more carefully at the benefits of truly professional nursing care. Without unlimited reimbursement possibilities, hospitals must look closely at the efficiency and effectiveness of their use of each category of employee. Employers may become more receptive to objective research that shows the overall benefits of paying professional nurses to provide professional nursing care.

Compared to Whom?

For a comparable worth argument to be complete, one must do more than explain the net benefits that nursing service provides. The point of the comparable worth argument is to find some kind of criteria outside the market for determining an adequate wage for nurses. Just knowing what nurses contribute does not satisfy that question. The issue of how they should be rewarded for what they contribute is still open. The comparable worth argument proposes that the criterion should be relational, i.e., that it should be made by comparing nursing with other occupations that provide the same amount of benefits, require comparable amounts of training, and have similar levels of accountability. It is not necessary that the other occupations be similar to nursing in the kind of benefit they provide or in the kinds of training and accountability demanded of them. What is necessary instead is a similarity in amount of such factors as education, experience, responsibility, analysis and decision-making, and contribution. The usual method of determining comparable worth is through some type of job evaluation. Jobs to be analyzed are described in terms of such factors, which are assigned a point value. The total scores for each job are used to group "comparable" jobs. It is expected that jobs within each point group would receive comparable wages. Jobs held mainly by women are underpaid if their wages are significantly lower than jobs of the same point value held predominantly by men.

THE MARKET FOR NURSING

A market is a basic model used for economic analysis. Economic analysis is a theoretical approach that categorizes and discusses human interactions in terms of buying and selling transactions. There are different kinds of markets. A free market exists when buyers and sellers have maximum freedom to determine what things (and how much of them) will be produced, bought, and sold and at what price they will be purchased. Among American economists it is commonly believed that a free market or free enterprise system is the best form of marketplace.

A free market creates an incentive to produce goods at the lowest possible cost. Consumers, when offered a choice, will seek to get maximum benefit from their purchases. Producers will always attempt to keep their costs as low as possible, for in a free market they must constantly compete against other producers seeking to offer similar products to the consumer at lower prices. A rational consumer who has a choice will ordinarily choose to pay less for the same item. Thus, producers are rewarded by consumers for producing what consumers will buy and doing it at the lowest possible cost. The result is that a maximum amount of products will be available at the lowest possible price, satisfying both consumers and the producers who serve them.

The relationship of quantity supplied to quantity demanded determines the price for which products are sold. If consumer demand is high and supply limited, suppliers can increase their prices and consumers will still purchase the item. At some point, however, the price of the item will exceed its value to the consumer; at that point, the consumer will no longer purchase at the increased price. Decreased purchasing will result in more of the commodity being available. In other words, it increases the supply. Supply is also increased when producers make more of the commodity. When supply exceeds demand, consumers will seek the lowest available price. A supplier, eager to sell an oversupply of the item, will reduce prices to encourage consumers to buy his product rather than a competitor's. Thus in a free market, theoretically, when supply exceeds demand, prices will fall; and when demand exceeds supply, prices for the commodity will rise. Under a free market model it is predictable that certain things will happen to nursing wages and the number of nurses in the labor force. In truth, the market for nursing cannot be adequately explained under a free market model.

In the market model, nurses are viewed as having a commodity for sale just as all other sellers do. That commodity is their professional services.

Their employers are the consumers of nursing services. This may sound a bit odd, but for most nurses, the patients whom they consider their clients are not the consumers of nursing care. Very few patients have the opportunity to decide how much nursing care they will purchase, what price they will be willing to pay for nursing care, and how much they will purchase. Patients are the recipients of nursing care, but in an economic sense, employers are the consumers of nursing labor.

The total number of nursing care hours that can be purchased at a given price is the supply of nursing labor. The demand for nursing labor is the amount that employers are willing to purchase at a given price. In a free market, if the price of nursing care is lowered, there will be a change in the quantity of it that consumers demand: at a lower price they will want to purchase more. But at the same time, at a lower price there will be a lesser quantity available for purchase. Fewer people will enter or remain in nursing; other occupations will become comparatively more attractive.

When there is a nursing shortage, the rewards of nursing at the present rate do not attract enough people into nursing. In a perfectly competitive market, employers will increase the amount of wages they will pay, and this will increase the number of nurses willing to sell their services. Current workers might choose to work longer hours, nurses not now working might re-enter the labor force, and people just now choosing a profession will find nursing an attractive choice. In a perfect market we would expect that as long as employers do not have enough nurses to meet their needs, wages would continue to rise and the number of people entering nursing would continue to grow. Conversely, if present wage levels attract enough nurses to meet employers' needs, they would not raise wages. If more than enough nurses are available at present wage levels, wages would drop in an open market and the number of nurses would begin to decline.

Thus, in a free market the prevailing wage would be the right wage. It would be right because any other wage level would draw either too many or too few nurses into the labor market. The model presumes that the buying and selling of services is done by people who have a free choice about how much to buy and sell. In examining the market for nursing, one sees that both the supply of and the demand for nursing services are caught in a set of constraints that this market model does not consider.

Because nursing is predominantly a women's profession, it is affected by the social constraints that affect women's lives. One of these constraints is that women have not traditionally been free to relocate and sell their professional services in other locations. When women marry and choose to have families, career moves involving geographic relocations are most often determined by the husband's professional situation rather than the wife's. Even if the woman desired to pursue her own career, relocation based on her career goals usually cannot be justified financially. Because women have traditionally earned less than their male counterparts, the financial security of the family has been primarily dependent upon the husband's income. Thus relocation decisions are most often dictated by the man's career path rather than the woman's.

Also, because hospitals have not traditionally competed with each other, they usually did not build in areas where one or more hospitals already existed. Most communities, other than large metropolitan areas, have only one or two hospitals. Thus, most nurses find themselves geographically restricted to one or two potential employers. The result is that a nurse dissatisfied with wages cannot freely change employers. Nurses are not as free as are producers and consumers in a perfect, free market. The supply of nursing services within a given community is therefore fairly stable and predictable, regardless of the level of wages offered.

Another factor that affects the supply of nursing services is related to the definition of nursing. We saw in Chapter 1 a definition of nursing that seems intelligible and correct to someone who already knows what nursing is. But, as we noted there, the real problem is to define nursing in such a way that it is informative to those who do not already understand. The nursing profession has failed to define what it contributes to patient care and to do so in such a way that patients and administrators know what nursing is and does.

Patients in hospitals can identify their nurses and can often identify tasks that nurses perform. But they also see aides and practical nurses performing many of the same tasks and may not be able to distinguish these different levels of care. When the patient receives the bill for his hospital care, there is no way for him to identify the nursing care he has received and what part of his bill it comprises. The cost of nursing care is typically hidden in the daily room charge along with such components as meals, housekeeping, and linen charges.

Efforts made to distinguish what nurses do by simple observation of the tasks they perform overlook the other patient needs that are attended to during the procedure and what might be the outcomes of two different approaches to the same task. Completion of tasks is not by itself an adequate measure of what professional nursing contributes to health care; it must be coupled with some measure of the outcome for the patient. The care and advocacy for the patient are, after all, part of what distinguishes truly professional nursing. The inability to identify what is different about professional nursing makes it difficult to determine what the supply of professional nurses is in relation to the roles in which they function. Thus, we might reasonably claim that there is not a defined market for professional nursing care. Even the administrator who hires the nurse is not always aware of the nature of the product and may not distinguish it from other kinds of labor and services.

This lack of differentiation results in "substitutability," which is the use of more than one level of personnel to carry out the same functions. When it appears that a different type of employee with a lower wage level can accomplish the same task, an employer will naturally tend to choose the lower wage level. This seems perfectly reasonable if we assume that the additional cost of hiring the higher-level employee yields no additional benefit; it is money wasted. The use of a licensed practical nurse as charge nurse on the night shift is one example of this. Hospitals have the freedom to make such substitutions and still receive reimbursement for nursing expenses. The patient is charged the same rate, regardless of the level of personnel responsible for his care.

Correlatively, nurses are sometimes used as substitutes for transporters, ward clerks, or laboratory technicians, taking on tasks for which these other groups are trained and hired. As a result, the wages of nurses are determined in part by the market for transporters, secretaries, or whatever group for which nurses are being substituted. The overall result of the muddy waters that presently surround the definition of nursing is that it is difficult to identify exactly what commodity nurses are selling and the benefits to the consumer of purchasing that commodity.

The Demand for Nursing Services

The demand for nursing is also complicated by the fact that the primary consumers of nursing services are employers rather than the direct recipients of nursing care. The largest employers of nurses are hospitals. Thus, the demand for nursing services is primarily determined by hospitals. Hospitals traditionally have not competed against each other for the purchase of available nursing services. In fact, there was little competition of any kind in the health care system until the 1980's. Hospital officials usually know about wage levels at other hospitals. But until very recently that knowledge was used mostly to ensure that no employer paid above the going rate.

As a result, the market does not function as it is expected to in a free market model; a shortage of workers will not necessarily bring an increase in wages. Purchasers gain power in a market whenever they cooperate with rather than compete against one another. These conditions result in an *oligopsonistic* market, a market in which fewer workers are hired and at lower prices than in a competitive market. The term oligopsonistic refers to a market in which there are only a few very powerful purchasers.

Cost Containment and the Demand for Nursing

In the 1980's, the increasing cost of health care has concerned individual consumers as well as third-party payors and health providers. There have been a number of responses, and a great deal of speculation has been heard about the long-term effects of these responses on health care delivery. Two specific responses merit attention in regard to their potential implications for nursing.

One is the change in the way third-party payors reimburse providers of health care. When the federal government realized that Medicare expenditures had increased from $3 billion in 1967 to $30.8 billion in 1980, it decided to implement another form of payment, called *prospective payment*.

Under prospective payment, the third-party payor calculates beforehand a reasonable average cost for a given diagnosis. The payor reimburses exactly that amount, regardless of the actual costs of the health care provider. If the providers' costs are greater than the reimbursement, they lose money. However, if providers can find a way to reduce costs below the amount of the reimbursement, they stand to gain. The system is now being implemented in phases throughout the United States. It used a method of classifying patients according to medical diagnosis in order to determine an appropriate amount of reimbursement. The classification system now being used is a *diagnosis-related grouping*, commonly known as DRG. The hospital is reimbursed the same amount for all patients classified in the same DRG. It is likely that the classification system will undergo refinement and change.

Private insurance companies are now watching the Medicare prospective payment system to determine whether to adopt some form of it themselves. In the meantime, they are experimenting with a variety of cost-reduction measures, such as utilization review, health maintenance organizations, and preferred provider arrangements.

The opportunity to make a profit by offering low-cost health care has led to another important change in health care in the U.S. that may have important ramifications for nursing. This is the stronger involvement of for-profit organizations in what was formerly a not-for-profit market. In 1982, 14 per cent of hospitals were owned by investors. A recent study commissioned by the American College of Hospital Administrators (1984) projected that by 1995 more than 23 per cent will be investor-owned. Investors have become involved in and have stimulated the growth of new endeavors such as urgent-care centers, home health care agencies, health maintenance organizations and nursing homes. Even not-for-profit organizations seek to create a dollar surplus that they will eventually put back into their organizations. The introduction of the profit-making component into health care delivery has stimulated competition among health care providers. Competition creates even greater incentives to keep costs down.

The increased emphasis on competition and cost containment can have both good and bad effects. As noted earlier, there are potential benefits to an open competitive market system: both buyers and sellers are free to do as they choose. There are incentives to provide the products that people most need and to do so at minimal costs. Obviously, waste in health care should be avoided and our available resources should be spent in ways that provide the maximum health benefit. In fact, traditional hospital accounting did not even enable hospitals to identify where their costs were incurred or how they could be reduced. As long as providers had the luxury of knowing that they would be reimbursed for all the care actually provided, they did not have to deal with the conflict between optimal care and cost containment. Current funding changes should curb unnecessary costs that were tolerated in the previous system.

However, in a competitive market, there is a danger that the needs of patients and clients will not be given the highest consideration when the provider firm must show a profit to satisfy its stockholders. To make money, organizations may be inclined to offer services that are lucrative rather than those for which there is a great need among persons who cannot afford to pay. Patients whose conditions require high concentrations of intense nursing care may not be desirable patients from a profit-making perspective. Even a well-intended provider can lose considerable money by providing appropriate care for a patient who requires an unusual intensity of care compared with others in the same diagnostic grouping.

Because nursing wages represent one of the largest components of hospital expenditures, administrators may attempt to hold wages down or reduce total numbers of nursing staff. Nurses may be faced with employment situations that offer what they consider unsatisfactory compensation. They must attempt to balance their concern for personal economic welfare with their professional commitment to act in the best interests of their patients. The next chapter examines more closely how nurses attempt to do this.

AN ASSESSMENT

The preceding discussion illustrates that there is no easy answer to the question of what constitutes an adequate wage for nurses. The performance of the marketplace itself is likely to give an unreliable answer, because of the imperfections identified earlier. Using comparable worth may provide some way of showing substantively the patterns of wage inequality in women's occupations. But the use of the comparable worth criterion assumes that it is possible to assess objectively what nurses contribute. The results of this are contingent upon both nursing's ability to specify its role with adequate precision and the success of nursing research in showing the outcomes of nursing care. It also depends on similar objective knowledge about the occupations to which nursing compares itself. Moreover, the comparisons fall on deaf ears unless they are successfully used to change administrative policy, to bring about legislation, or to convince the courts.

Comparable worth, even if it can be implemented, is not a panacea. If it is intended to provide a one-time correction in wages, the danger is that once wages of comparable occupations are equalized, the same forces that made them unequal will eventually return us to past inequities. All the same forces that made the market for nursing labor an imperfect market could emerge again.

On the other hand, if nurses assume that mechanisms such as the comparable worth argument are to be used indefinitely, they are cutting themselves off from possible advantages of a free market.

WHERE NEXT?

The discussion of economic issues in nursing has described the market for nursing's services within a changing health care delivery system. It has pointed out some of the reasons why the supply and demand for nursing services do not interact in the way one would expect in a free marketplace, and identified some of the things nurses are doing to clarify the contribution of nursing to overall patient care. These efforts are necessary in order to establish the true value of nursing care. The concept of comparable worth is one mechanism for trying to establish the value of traditionally female occupations in relation to male-dominated occupations requiring equivalent degrees of skill, education, and experience. Overall, it has been suggested that nurses are not adequately compensated for the contribution that they make to patient care, and that nurses are not and probably should not be content with their current wages.

How, then, does the individual nurse deal with this problem? How can professional nurses reconcile their desire for better wages with their professional commitment to their patients? Does it run counter to the spirit of professionalism to demand higher wages and possibly drive up the costs of health care?

Increasing the cost of health care in the present environment is likely to result in reduced amount or quality of care available. Nurses can no longer be sure that wage increases will come from raising rates or reducing profits. In many cases, surpluses no longer exist. In other cases, administrators face an uncertain future and are reluctant to overextend their resources. Also, providers are not as free to raise rates as they once were. Thus demands for higher wages may be met by the hiring of fewer nurses at the higher wage or the substitution of less qualified personnel to provide nursing services.

It was pointed out early in the chapter that, if we accept as a basic ethical principle that all persons have the right to protect their own welfare, then nurses do have the right to adequate compensation for their work. The challenge is to reconcile this moral right to pursue one's personal welfare with the moral duty that professionals have to their patients. That duty must be understood in the environment in which it occurs. At the present, that environment is complex and uncertain.

In the current environment, it is easy to view the best interests of patients and the economic interests of nurses as irreconcilably in conflict. But it can be argued that the pursuit of increased wages can also further the professional commitment that nurses make to serve their patients. This belief is summed concisely in the Code for Nurses:

> The nurse participates in the profession's efforts to establish and maintain conditions of employment conducive to high quality nursing care.

The same statement goes on to specify that nurses must be concerned with terms and conditions of employment that are conducive to high quality nursing care.

The Code appears to consider two reasons for the need to address compensation as one of the "terms of employment conducive to high quality care." These are the actual and the symbolic value of compensation.

Economic incentives attract qualified personnel. To the extent that nursing wages rise, recruits will be attracted to nursing who may otherwise have been drawn to other occupations for economic reasons. Competent nurses will be less likely to leave nursing for other well-paying opportunities. From this standpoint, adequate compensation is essential to maintaining high quality professional services because it helps ensure that persons entering the field are among the brightest and the best. But the economic status of nurses as a group also affects the professional influence of individual practitioners and their ability to fulfill their professional commitment.

The compensation that one receives is a symbol of professional power. Professional power is the measure of autonomy, the ability to control one's own practice and to participate in decision-making and policy formation. Professional power enables nurses to exert influence over the work environment, the conditions under which they provide professional services. Individual nurses do not gain influence solely on the basis of their own knowledge and skills. Part of their professional power stems from the generalized perceptions that others hold of the nursing profession. Perceptions of power and influence are based on numerous factors, one of which is wealth (Korda, 1975). Money, then, is a source of power for its direct uses and also for the image of professional influence it helps to create.

It should be noted that increased money and power do not necessarily draw into the profession only those ready and able to make a professional commitment. They can attract also those who are interested primarily in money and power. Thus the argument that adequate compensation is necessary for the fulfillment of the nursing commitment can be a dangerous one. One must understand that adequate compensation is a necessary condition for the exercise of professional autonomy. Professional autonomy includes the policing of members of the profession, so that those who are not ready to commit themselves to the goals of the profession are not allowed to remain members solely for the money and power they can achieve.

SUMMARY

Owing to several factors, nurses have not received the level of compensation that persons in positions of similar responsibility would receive or that they would have received in an open marketplace. This raises the question of fairness to nurses, but it also raises questions about the long-term ability of the profession to meet the duties of its professional commitment. In the present environment it is uncertain what professional nurses can ethically do. However, there are ways in which nurses are working together in efforts to improve the economic situation of the profession. In the next chapter, we will look more closely at collective action within the profession and nurses' efforts to meet their professional responsibilities to their patients.

For Further Discussion

1. One of the results of the prospective payment system is that average length of patient hospital stay has been reduced. What are some potential problems associated with earlier discharge for patients? How might such situations create ethical concerns for the nurses caring for these patients? What would you do if a patient for whom you were caring was to be discharged sooner than you believed to be safe? What are some possible approaches to dealing with this type of situation?

2. Research the methods used to compare jobs and establish comparable worth. Try to apply these methods to a comparison of nursing with other job categories within the hospital setting, such as pharmacist, physician, physical therapist, and dietitian. How does nursing compare with these other groups in regard to such criteria as skill, effort, responsibility, working conditions, and education required by the job? How does nursing compare to these other categories in terms of wages?

3. Consider the discussion about the supply and demand for nursing services and the factors that affect these two. Are there any measures open to the profession that would affect the supply of nurses? What actions have been taken by other professions to exert control over the supply of practitioners? What, if any, are the ethical implications of such actions?

Bibliography

Aiken, L. (1982). Statistical Profile of Today's Nurses. In Nursing in the 1980's: Crises, Opportunities and Challenges. Philadelphia: J. B. Lippincott Company.

Alessi, D. J. (1983). Proving Sex-Based Wage Discrimination Under Federal Law. Kansas City, Missouri: American Nurses Association.

American College of Hospital Administrators (1984). Health Care in the 1990's: Trends and Strategies. Chicago: The College.

American Hospital Association (1984). Hospital Statistics, 1984 Edition. Chicago: The Association.

American Journal of Nursing News Item about comparable worth (1983).

American Nurses Association (1976). Code for Nurses with Interpretive Statements. Kansas City, Missouri: The Association.

Appeals Court Overturns Ruling on Comparable Worth. (1985). American Nurse, 17(9):9, October.

Brennan v. Owensboro-Davies City Hospital. (6th Circuit, 1975), N0.73-1261, 10EPD para 19,404.

Brett, J. L. (1983). How Much Is a Nurse's Job Really Worth? American Journal of Nursing, 83(6):877-881.

Bullough, B. (1978). The Struggle for Women's Rights in Denver: A Personal Account. Nursing Outlook, 26:566.

Bunzel, J. H. (1981). To Each According to Her Worth? The Public Interest, 77-93.

Curtin, L. (1983). Determining Cost of Nursing Services per DRG. Nursing Management, 14:16-20.

Grimaldi, P. L. and Micheletti, J. A. (1982). DRG Reimbursement: RIM's and the Cost of Nursing Care. Nursing Management, 13:12-22.

Kim, M. J., McFarland, G. K. and McLane, A. M. (1984). Classification of Nursing Diagnoses: Proceedings of the Fifth National Conference. St.Louis: C. V. Mosby Company.

Korda, M. (1975). Power: How to Get It, How to Use It. New York: Random House.

Krueoff, C. (1980). Money: The Question of Men, Women, and Comparable Worth. In Grune, J. A., editor (1980). Manual of Pay Equity: Raising Wages for Women's Work. Washington, D.C.: Conference Publications.

Lemon v. City of Denver, 22FEP Cases 959 (10th Cir.)

Livernash, E. R., (1980). Comparable Worth: Issues and Alternatives. Washington, D.C.: Equal Employment Advisory Council.

McCarty, P. (1985). Commission Rejects Comparable Worth, Blames Socialization. The American Nurse, 17(5):1.

Mitchell, M., Miller, J., Welches, L., and Walker, D. (1984). Determining Cost of Direct Nursing Care by DRG's. Nursing Management, 15(4):29.

Prescott, P. (1986). DRG Prospective Reimbursement: The Nursing Intensity Factor. Nursing Management, 17(1):43.

Ratner, R. S. (1980). Equal Employment Policy for Women. Philadelphia: Temple University Press.

Remick, H. (1980). Beyond Equal Pay for Equal Worth: Comparable Worth in the State of Washington. In Equal Employment Policy for Women: Strategies for Implementation in the United States, Canada and Western Europe. Ratner, R. S., editor (1980). Philadelphia: Temple University Press.

Rothman, N. and Rothman, D. (1980). Equal Pay for Comparable Work. Nursing Outlook, 28:728.

Thaker, H. H. (1983). Wage Setting and Evaluation: Economic Principles for Registered Nurses. Kansas City, Missouri: American Nurses Association.

Trofino, J. (1985). RIMs: Skirting the Edge of Disaster. Nursing Management, 16(7):48.

U.S. Bureau of Census (1985). Statistical Abstract of the United States: 1986. (106th Ed.) Washington, D.C.

Weingard, M. (1984). Establishing Comparable Worth Through Job Evaluation. Nursing Outlook, 32(2):110.

Chapter Nine

COLLECTIVE ACTION

We have emphasized throughout this book that persons entering the profession of nursing accept dual responsibilities. They are responsible first of all to the clients for whom they provide direct nursing care. Second, by identifying themselves as members of a profession, individual nurses accept the collective responsibilities that accompany the profession's commitment to society at large.

Maintaining their own expertise and meeting the obligations of their individual relationships with clients are ways that nurses can help ensure that their individual professional responsibilities are met. But individual competence and integrity are not enough. Professionalism also demands awareness of and participation in activities essential to the full expression of nursing's contract with society, even if they seem irrelevant to the delivery of direct bedside care. These activities relate to the collective responsibilities of the profession, those responsibilities that cannot be met by the actions of one or a few nurses. These obligations can be accomplished only when members of the group are involved in coordinated efforts to meet mutually accepted goals.

Most policies and decisions affecting nursing practice are made with more than one individual nurse in mind. Policy-makers deal with nurses as a group rather than as individuals. This is true at the institutional level and also at the broader level of social policy. Decisions that affect large numbers of people are not made on the basis of the individual commitments, preferences, and considerations of each person involved. As an example, if the administrators of a nursing service department are considering the implementation of primary nursing, they must take many factors into account. They look at the impact of primary nursing on the care delivered to patients. They consider the reactions of nursing and non-nursing caregivers. They consider the financial impact of such a change. They analyze the impact of this new form of patient care delivery on such indirect factors as staff development costs, secretarial support services, and staffing patterns. Although individual preferences and goals may be considered, ultimately such a decision is based on the overall goals of the institution and the nursing department for which the nurses work.

Certain goals common to all nurses in the department will be met if the decision made is consistent with departmental and overall institutional goals. When a nurse accepts a position in a particular institution, she is tacitly accepting the goals of the institution and the nursing department. Thus, if a policy decision is made on the basis of consideration of these common goals, it should also be compatible with the individual's personal professional goals. The decision to adopt primary nursing as the most effective way to meet the goals of care as they are expressed in the institution should be acceptable to individual practitioners in the nursing department.

Not all individuals may be comfortable with such a decision. One nurse may think that primary nursing still does not offer the autonomy desired or needed for professional practice. Others may believe that they cannot accept the additional responsibility inherent in primary nursing. Those nurses who are exceptions face the challenge of addressing the conflicts between institutional goals and their own personal goals. Often such differences are more perceived than real and can be resolved fairly easily. There is, of course, always the possibility that the conflict cannot be resolved between what practitioners believe they need to meet their professional commitment and what the institutional environment offers. A practitioner may even find it necessary to seek a different environment in which to practice. Such considerations are part of a nurse's decisions about how and where to practice, which were discussed in Chapter 5. If a number of individual nurses are uncomfortable with an institutional decision, they are much more likely to influence the decision-making process if they approach their nursing administrator as a group rather than as individuals.

Collective efforts such as this at the institutional level may directly affect the nurse's individual practice. Efforts to influence social policy have more far-reaching and often indirect effects on patient care. In the larger social context, nurses, as are other professional and occupational groups, are treated as groups rather than as individuals. Governmental policies and laws are made on the basis of the common goals and commitment expressed by the professional group rather than on consideration of individual practitioners. When there are groups within the profession expressing differing goals, policy makers frequently base their decisions on the needs or viewpoints of the most vocal or visible group. They are still dealing with groups of nurses rather than individuals. Individual nurses who wish to make their concerns known can most effectively do so through the group. Changes in nurse practice acts, for example, are best accomplished by groups of nurses working closely with legislators rather than by each practitioner attempting to work as an individual to influence the legislative process.

Nurses not only practice in a social context, they realize that their clients live and function in a social context. Their concern for the health of their clients reaches beyond the immediate environment in which they provide direct nursing service. They also want to promote the type of society in which their clients can experience healthy and fulfilling lives, whether or not they require direct nursing care. Nursing as a profession seeks to use its knowledge and expertise to affect social policies relating to health and those factors that impinge upon it. This kind of influence can be exerted through representation on policy-making boards and committees or in government agencies. Such activities may not have an immediate and perceptible effect on individual nursing practice, but they are essential for fulfilling the broad general commitment that the profession has made to society as a whole. These activities can be carried out only when individual nurses take part in them as part of their acceptance of the collective commitment of the profession.

The collective responsibilities of the profession, then, exist because the profession exists and because its members have made a special commitment to society. Collective responsibilities require group or collective action in order to meet them. Collective action is also necessary in many situations in order to ensure that individual professionals can meet their commitments to direct client care, since collective efforts generate the necessary influence to alter the practice environment. We have cited several examples of collective activity among nurses and numerous others could be identified. Generally, however, collective efforts fall into one of three broad categories, which we will discuss more fully. One is political activity, in the form of participation in the governmental process; another, the influence of the professional association, a special form of collective activity characteristic of professional groups.

A third type of collective activity in which nurses are becoming increasingly involved is *collective bargaining*. Closely associated with collective bargaining is the strike, perhaps the ultimate form of collective action. The strike poses a dilemma for the professional because it creates a conflict between individual professional responsibilities and collective responsibilities as a member of a professional group. We will address each of these forms of collective activity.

COLLECTIVE ACTIVITY AND LEGISLATIVE ACTION

One of the distinctive features of American society is the manner in which individual citizens can participate in the political process. Individuals can express their opinions about issues and candidates by exercising their right to vote. They have relatively easy access to lawmakers and policy makers and can make their individual needs known to those who make major social and political decisions. Ideally any individual can influence the nation's laws and policies by expressing his or her needs to those in policy-making positions.

Theoretically then, the needs or problems of any one individual can influence the actions of top-level administrators in public or private institutions. In reality, this rarely happens. Isolated incidents can be cited when special legislation was introduced to solve some individual's unusual or particularly difficult problems. But more often than not, the individual who influences policy decisions does so through some form of group activity.

Policies are deliberately chosen courses of action directed toward the achievement of a goal or the resolution of a problem. They are typically developed through some form of joint decision-making process, such as committees or the legislative branch of government. Policies address group concerns or issues rather than narrow individual problems. Social policies address the social structure or environment in which we live and work. They serve to create that environment, so to speak. If we are dissatisfied with the social environment in which we find ourselves, we must initiate the appropriate action to alter that environment. Realistically that means that we must identify other individuals who share our concern and work together to create change.

The environment in which nurses practice is shaped most directly by policies of the institution in which they deliver nursing care. To influence such policies, nurses must work together. When individual nurses unite for common goals and concerns and work through their representatives on key policy-making committees, they are exerting an influence in decision-making that they would not have as individuals.

But policies and laws originating in the broader health care delivery system and society as a whole will also affect the environment in which nursing care is provided. Professional practitioners attempt to alter policies outside their immediate work settings that inhibit or enhance their practice. Because policies at all levels typically address group concerns, the individual nurse will have limited success in creating policy change. That is because policy makers are most receptive to the informed views of groups of people or organizations rather than the opinions of individuals. The most effective way for nurses to influence social policy decisions is through some form of collective or group effort. The actions of individuals are still necessary, but if those individuals are speaking or acting as representatives of a professional organization or group, their efforts will have greater impact.

The need for organized group efforts to influence legislative policy has been recognized by nurses since the inception of modern nursing in this country. The first state nurses' associations were organized for the express purpose of unifying to influence the passage of licensure laws in each state.

However, as a whole the profession has not recognized the full potential of collective political activity until recent years. By exerting their collective influence, nurses have made their concerns known to policymakers and frequently have had a major impact on political outcomes. Let's look at an example of how nurses' collective political efforts have influenced legislation when individual efforts would likely have failed.

The Nurse Training Act Recisions

In November 1978, legislation authorizing continuation of the nurse training funds for the 1979–1980 fiscal year was passed by both houses of Congress and sent to President Carter for his signature. Carter vetoed the bill by neglecting to sign it into law. In January 1979, Carter proposed a recision of additional nurse training monies. Money to be rescinded had already been allocated and included in institutional budgets to provide operating funds and student financial aid (American Journal of Nursing, Jan., 1979). The sudden reduction in funding created an immediate financial crisis for many schools of nursing across the country.

Nurses across the country, concerned about the effect funding cuts would have on education and practice, initiated a number of collective responses to President Carter's decisions. Representatives of four major nursing organizations, the American Nurses' Association, the National League for Nursing, the American Association of Colleges of Nursing, and the National Student Nurses' Association, held a news conference and discussed their concerns about the funding cuts and their beliefs about the impact on the supply of registered nurses. In New York City representatives from 35 nursing organizations and other health groups formed the "Committee to Save the Nurse Training Act," and at a rally of 500 people announced that the purpose of the committee was to mobilize one million nurses to contact the White House concerning the bill. In Maryland, the deans of the state's seven baccalaureate nursing programs held a press conference to discuss the implications of the veto. In addition to the open expressions of concern, nursing representatives also inundated Congressional representatives with empirical data refuting the President's claim that there was no shortage of nurses at that time across the country (American Journal of Nursing, Feb. and March, 1979).

These events represented a cohesive response by many groups of nurses to one particular presidential policy. The result of their efforts was that in March 1979, both houses of Congress approved a change in the amount of rescinded funds. A new version of the Nurse Training Act was subsequently reintroduced into Congress and passed.

This example illustrates how nurses working together can influence legislation and policy, even when it might appear that a decision has been finalized. Individual nurses' views on the legislation for nurse training funds may have had some influence on the vote of some legislators. But even thousands of nurses, acting as individuals, would not have had the same impact as 500 rallying and making a unified statement, or seven speaking as representatives of professional organizations. Policy makers and legislators must function within the context of group interests and concerns; they pay greatest heed to voices that represent group interests and concerns. Unified efforts have an impact that individual efforts simply will not have.

THE PROFESSIONAL ASSOCIATION

One form of collective endeavor that is characteristic of the professions is the professional association. A professional association is an organization of practitioners who have banded together to perform social functions that they cannot perform as separate individuals. Typically, professional associations emerge early in the development of a new profession (Goode, 1957). Practitioners recognize their common concerns and interests and are moved to organize around them. In nursing, for example, the founders of the first nursing organizations were drawn together by their common concerns about quality of care and the poor preparation of many nurses. They joined together to work for reforms that they could not have accomplished as individuals.

The presence of a strong professional association is beneficial in a number of ways. The long-term benefactors of the association's activities are the recipients of nursing care. The maintenance and continued improvement of nursing care is the ultimate purpose for which the professional association exists. The association provides benefits for individual members as well as for the profession as a whole.

Individual Benefits

Typically, membership in a professional association is limited to those persons with a certain expertise. This distinguishes the experts from the nonexperts and sets them apart from the general population. This separation provides a certain prestige. The association also provides practitioners with the moral and social support to help them perform their roles as professionals. A bond, rising out of their common commitment to the clients they serve, develops among members of the profession and is fostered through the association. Each is expected to live up to or exceed the acceptable standards set by the profession and to see to it that others do so also.

But colleagues do not merely monitor one another's competence. They also support one another and provide the sustained motivation that is necessary to continually perform at one's best. The association provides opportunities for practitioners to share expertise and collaborate on practice and research endeavors. These kinds of exchanges stimulate professional growth of individual practitioners and serve to continually upgrade the knowledge and expertise upon which good nursing care is based. Thus the direct benefits to the practitioner also enhance the profession as a whole and result in the benefit to the clients of continually improved nursing care.

A professional association also recognizes individual excellence through certification and award programs. This kind of recognition from an organized group of one's professional peers stimulates continued excellence in individual practice and provides a sense of satisfaction in knowing that one is doing well.

Benefits to the Profession

Other aspects of the association contribute most directly to the fulfillment of the collective obligations of the profession, and benefits to the individual member are less evident. The professional association provides a visible, formally organized mechanism through which members can work together to accomplish goals that they could not accomplish alone. It provides the structure and support for group endeavors, which must take place if the profession is to meet its collective commitment to society. For example, an essential obligation of the profession is to establish and monitor standards of education, practice, and research. This must be done with input from as many individual practitioners as possible. The standards accepted by the profession must represent the views of the members of the profession. The professional association provides a mechanism, although an imperfect one, for a flow of information from individual practitioners to the leaders who formulate the standards and communicate them to society.

One function of the professional association is to constantly press for higher standards within the profession in anticipation of future changes in the profession's relationship with society. The standards it sets must be more exacting than those that the lay public might require. Members of the profession are the true experts who realize the potentialities for improved services, and they must strive to develop those potentialities. The association stimulates individual members to not simply be content with what is but to be looking to the future and preparing for it.

We have already discussed the importance of research and the development of knowledge to a profession. The specialized knowledge underlying its practice is the mechanism through which the profession meets its obligations to its clients. The professional association has the function of advancing research through funding of agencies or individual researchers and also acting as a clearinghouse for professional knowledge. Professional meetings and publications sponsored by the association facilitate the dissemination and sharing of research and knowledge.

The professional association also defines and enforces rules of professional conduct. In this sense it functions as the collective conscience of the profession. The code of conduct developed through the association is a reflection of the profession's understanding of its commitment to clients and society. Interpretations of the professional code of ethics or analyses of particularly complex or troublesome ethical dilemmas often come from the professional association.

A profession relates to other professions and organized groups through its official organization. The association acts as the official voice of the profession in political and legislative activities. It is the organ through which nurses can have dialogues with other professions on such matters as health care delivery, issues of higher education, or interprofessional relationships. This kind of representation is more than just a group effort, because it comes through a group composed exclusively of experts from the profession and recognized as the custodian of the profession's goals and ideals.

The professional association serves several necessary functions in the business of the profession. Many of these functions cannot be carried out by nurses as individuals. They are most effectively executed through a formal organization composed of experts in the profession and recognized by society as an official voice of the group. The individual who joins the professional association recognizes that the group can accomplish more than individuals, and that group goals are accomplished through the actions of individuals. The individual member receives direct and indirect benefits from the association but is also contributing to the accomplishment of collective professional goals.

The Many Organizations of Nursing

In the previous discussion we have referred to the professional association. We have assumed a distinction between a professional association and professional organizations. A *professional association* is an organization of practitioners who are motivated to join together because of common interests flowing from their professional commitment. Membership in professional associations is limited to persons who share the expertise of the profession or perhaps are preparing to enter the profession. The professional association speaks for the profession as a whole and is recognized by society as the voice of the profession. One of its primary functions is to establish and enforce standards of professional conduct for ALL its members. The official professional association does not limit itself to issues and concerns of specific practice groups but rather serves as the guardian of standards for the profession as a whole.

Other professional organizations do not address the professional commitment with the same perspective as does the professional association. They typically develop as subgroups of the larger professional group. Subgroup interests may be functional, such as educational organizations or nurse researcher groups. Formal groups may organize around common clinical interests, such as oncology nurses or school nurses. Other clinical or practice organizations may develop around broader areas, such as gerontology or reality therapy, and include persons from many disciplines in their membership. Some, such as the National League for Nursing, whose major activities involve quality assurance, may include non-nurses.

Nursing has always had more than one strong professional organization. The first formal organization in the United States was the Society for Superintendents of Training Schools, which later became the National League for Nursing. The NLN has always had nursing education as its primary focus. Although the association is actively involved in furthering the goals of the profession in general, it is primarily a quality assurance agency whose major purpose is to credential educational programs (see Editor's note in Sleicher, 1981). Its membership includes both nurses and non-nurses who share its goals.

The second formal nursing organization in the United States, the Nurses' Associated Alumnae of the United States and Canada, was started in 1896 and became the American Nurses' Association in 1911. The objectives of this first association for trained nurses were to establish and maintain a code of ethics, to elevate the standard of nursing education, and to promote the usefulness and honor of the profession and its financial and other interests (Flanagan, 1976). The goals of this organization remain essentially the same today.

Throughout the years many organizations have developed around specialty interests. One particularly strong group during the early part of the century was that of the public health nurses, who maintained their separate organization until 1952, at which time they were absorbed into the NLN. The strongest specialty organization in the 1980's is the American Association of Critical Care Nurses, whose membership is exceeded only by the ANA and the NLN. It was this organization that was instrumental in organizing the Federation of Specialty Nursing Organizations and ANA in 1973 to promote cooperation among specialty groups and the American Nurses' Association (ANA, 1980).

All of these different professional groups serve important functions. One of the most important is the collective effort discussed throughout this chapter—the approach to problem-solving that accomplishes outcomes that individual actions will not. They also provide opportunities for practitioners to communicate with others who share their interests and problems and to seek common solutions that will ultimately benefit the recipients of their professional services.

There is a danger, however, in having so many different professional groups: the power in numbers that accounts for the success of group efforts becomes diffused throughout so many different groups that it is lost. This is particularly detrimental when the purposes of various groups are not clearly understood by the members, and membership in one or more of the many specialty groups is substituted for membership in the professional association.

All nurses share a similar professional commitment. There is a need for a far-reaching organization that encompasses all professional concerns of nurses and that relates to the society they serve. Because of the breadth of such a mission, it is not likely that a professional association will satisfy all practitioners all the time. Yet the need for a professional association is great enough that it is important to maintain one's active affiliation and to use the association to achieve professional goals. The alternative is to go it alone; to attempt to do so shows a lack of awareness of the social forces that affect one's ability to practice nursing professionally.

COLLECTIVE ACTION AND UNIONIZATION

Professional associations and labor unions are usually different kinds of organizations, though both serve as focal points for collective action. Unions ordinarily take on issues faced by a specific employment group in their relationship with a specific employer. Professional associations, on the other hand, deal with broader issues related to the whole profession and its ability to practice professionally. This distinction should not be taken as absolute, for both kinds of organization have sometimes become involved in issues related to the other.

One of the most important and notable functions of a union is to represent employees in negotiation of employment contracts with their employer, i.e., in collective bargaining. A restrictive set of laws prevented the development of collective bargaining in health care at a time when there was significant union activity among the rest of the United States work force. In 1935 the National Labor Relations Act (NLRA) provided a protective framework for workers who formed unions and bargained collectively. At that time, health care institutions seem to have been included in the act, but there was little union activity in such institutions then. This may have been due in part to the fact that many nurses were working in private duty and public health nursing. The great growth of hospitals and the decline of private duty nursing did not occur until the 1940's and 1950's.

In 1947 the NLRA was amended by the Taft-Hartley Amendments, which specifically excluded hospital employees from the protections provided for workers attempting to organize. The growth of unions in hospitals was prevented by the lack of legal protection for employees who organized. The ANA immediately began working for the repeal of the Taft-Hartley Amendments (Kalisch and Kalisch, 1986). Through its Commission on Economic and General Welfare the professional association assisted state nurses' associations in their efforts to negotiate economic issues between practitioners and their employers. At the end of 1970, a total of 333 contracts negotiated by 32 state nurses' associations were in force for 40,000 nurses and 471 employers (Flanigan, 1976).

Public Law 93-360 of 1974, which repealed the Taft-Hartley Amendments, gave health care workers all the same union organizing rights as other workers, but it imposed some limitations on the right to strike in hospitals. Organizing activities by state nurses' associations and by trade unions not previously associated with nursing increased rapidly following the repeal of the Taft-Hartley Amendments (Bentivegna, 1979).

Unionization of professional nurses brings certain important benefits because it enables nurses to more effectively engage in collective action related to their immediate work situation. The professional duty to engage in collective action when necessary to uphold the professional commitment may very well require that nurses organize collectively not only at the state and national level but even within their own work places. But any claim about an ethical duty to join a union must be tempered with cautions: the unionization of health professionals raises some controversial issues that need to be examined.

Many of these controversial issues stem from the mixed identity experienced by individual professionals in union structures. For some of the more established professions, establishing or joining a union means a loss of the individual autonomy so highly prized in the professions. For nursing, however, which has never experienced that sort of autonomy, unionization does not present the same problem. Still, the similarities with labor unions can result in labor contracts that provide undeserved employment protection for incompetent nurses. They can create or perpetuate adversarial situations between staff nurses and administrative personnel in an institution. The idea of nurses being union employees in the same way as factory workers are unionized can lead to an image problem, with patients less ready to regard nurses as professionals.

Indeed, none of these things need necessarily happen. In fact, nurses have tried to avoid this by using their own professional associations as collective bargaining agents rather than relying on labor unions. A number of state nurses' associations currently serve as collective bargaining agents. In defense of this practice, we can say that it is more likely that the professional duties of nurses and the quality of patient care will be considered during negotiations when negotiators are sensitive to these professional concerns.

But there are some important drawbacks to using the professional association as a bargaining agent. First, it must be admitted that unionization with collective bargaining is still a somewhat controversial and divisive issue among nurses themselves. For nursing's professional association to undertake this function could put that divisiveness into the middle of the professional association, thereby making it less effective. Second, some nurses who want to be involved in their professional association are prevented from doing so when it becomes their bargaining agent. Nurses with administrative duties are not included in a bargaining unit, nor are members of a religious organization that sponsors a hospital in which they are employed.

The Strike as Tool

The legal right to engage in collective bargaining is by itself an empty right. A bargaining position is powerful only to the extent that it is coupled with the ability to offer the other party something desirable or to withhold something desirable. Withdrawal of professional services provides that power.

As employed professionals, nurses have a twofold relationship with patients. On one hand, they owe their patients nursing care because of an employment agreement with an employer. On the other hand, they owe care to patients because of their direct professional-client relationship with them. In an industrial setting, the refusal to work disrupts production and exposes the employer to a financial loss. Certainly, the absence of a nursing staff will prevent the hospital from earning revenue. In that respect, a strike at a hospital and a strike at a factory are similar. But the refusal to work may well conflict with ethical duties that professional nurses have to patients and that the hospital has to patients. This does not by itself indicate that a strike by professional nurses would be unethical. In Chapter 3 we showed through the examination of a case that all the duties and rights and all of the good things to do in a particular situation are not always compatible. In the strike situation, we must again look at the various moral values expressed in any decision before drawing final conclusions.

Striking nurses may well find themselves trying to choose among conflicting duties. It seems beyond question that professionals have duties not to abandon the clients with whom they already have a professional relationship. But we have argued throughout this volume that the ethical duties of a professional go beyond those of the immediate situation, i.e., that professionals both individually and collectively bear the responsibility for ensuring that they and their colleagues will in the future be able to live up to the professional commitment they have made.

A nurse may have to choose between fulfilling obligations for present patients and withholding professional services through a strike. When the strike is intended to solve professional problems and to make it possible to practice nursing more effectively, then the conflict is really between the duty to serve present patients and the duty to ensure continued ability to serve future patients. When continuing education benefits, staffing level, and other such quality of care issues are an important part of negotiations, it is likely that such a conflict is developing. The problem is to determine which duty one should observe when it is impossible both to serve present patients and to ensure quality of care in the future.

Care of present patients is a compelling moral duty for several reasons. First, they have a greater claim on the professional than do possible future patients; they are already in a professional-client relationship, which ought to be characterized by fidelity, trust, and good faith. Second, they are likely to be most immediately in need of care. So any claim that the welfare of present patients should be sacrificed for some future good would have to be based on some extremely important obligation or on some extraordinary improvement that would be gained. Whether that is so requires a thorough understanding of the situation at hand. Among the questions that would have to be resolved are the following:

1. What harm might be done to present patients and how likely is it that this harm would occur?
2. What improvements are expected as a result of the strike?
3. How likely is it that the strike will be successful in gaining those improvements?
4. How likely is it that the same improvements could be made without resorting to a strike?
5. What effect might the strike have on nurses' future ability to develop good faith relationships with patients?

If, after considering the facts of the case in relation to all these questions, one becomes convinced that a duty to strike exists, then the matter is not thereby settled. There is still a duty to see that present patients are cared for. When repeal of the Taft-Hartley Amendments in 1974 gave hospital employees the right to collective bargaining, legal restrictions on the right to strike were established so that patients would not suffer in labor disputes. Among them is a requirement that unions give a 10-day notification before a strike, in order to help hospitals make arrangements for patients who might be affected by the strike. In general, striking nurses have gone out of their way to see to it that present patients are adequately cared for. Often they continue to staff intensive care units, delivery rooms, and emergency rooms if other arrangements cannot be made for patients. In doing so they may be going beyond what the law requires of them, but professional ethics requires that patients not be abandoned, even when adequate notice is given.

What can be said of a strike by professionals for personal economic benefit? First, as we have pointed out in Chapter 8, it is unlikely that a strike for economic benefit would be a strike with only that objective. Attractive wages seem likely to result in competent practitioners, both in the short run and in the long run. A strike that is intended to serve the strikers' interests exclusively raises an important question for the professional. We argued in the last chapter that professionals (just as other people) have rights to personal welfare and have ethical duties to provide for their dependents. Can these rights and duties ever outweigh the duty of professionals to care for their present patients? In some extreme situations, perhaps they can. In making such a decision, one is not simply weighing one ethical value against another. Instead, one is rejecting the whole context of professionalism in favor of some other value system. There is nothing more to be said about professional ethics at that point, even if the rejection of the professional commitment is justifiable on some other basis.

In summary, to the extent that strikes by health professionals require refusal to care for present patients, they involve a violation of professional ethics. Although it is conceivable that some more compelling duty could justify a strike, the professional still has the duty to see that present patients are cared for rather than abandoned.

The Free Rider Issue

This chapter has discussed a variety of collective activities and their relations to professional ethics in nursing. Because the impact of collective activities on one's own daily professional practice is not always direct and immediate, it is possible to ignore them and still be convinced that one is truly practicing professional nursing. We have argued that for individuals to do so is to risk creating or perpetuating an environment hostile to the practice of truly professional nursing.

Sometimes the only way some public good can be provided is by extending its benefits both to those who pay for it and those who refuse to pay. (Street lights, paved streets, and public television stations are examples of items from whose benefits people are not easily excluded.) Free riders know that, even if they do not pay a share of the price, the benefit will still be provided. The inaction of one person is not enough to keep the benefit from being realized. When many people realize that there is nothing to prevent them from taking a free ride, not enough paying riders are left to create the benefit. If everyone who knew they could enjoy public television without paying for it chose not to pay, soon there would be no public television.

The problem of collective action in nursing is a sort of free rider problem: the creation of the kind of environment in which it is possible for nurses to honor the professional commitment they have made is a benefit to those nurses; it makes it possible for them to do what they have promised to do. But that good can be provided only if nurses act collectively. It is possible for the individual nurse to abstain from collective action, pretending that her or his own professional life occurs in a vacuum. In doing so, the nurse is taking a free ride. When large numbers of nurses choose to act in this way, nursing as a profession becomes an illusion in our society.

For Further Discussion

1. Public Law 93-630 (the repeal of the Taft-Hartley Amendments) offers an

alternative for the nurse who in good conscience refuses to join a union. Such a nurse in a unionized hospital must contribute an amount equivalent to the union dues to a charity acceptable to both the hospital and the union. Discuss this. What problem is it attempting to resolve? Does it do so? Does the nurse who chooses this alternative solve the free rider problem? Are there other forms of collective action available for a nurse who finds unionization unethical?

2. List and explain some ways that a nurse can use to determine if there is a strong enough certainty that there is no way other than a strike to improve the quality of care; that the demand for which the strike is called will have the desired effect on quality of care.

3. Look back at the discussion of the Nurse Training Act case. Use it to trace how collective activities of this nature can determine the conditions within which the individual nurse practices. How would this particular situation affect practice with and without the disputed funding?

4. Consider your experiences in nursing school. Identify situations in which group or collective action by students did have or could have had influence in decision-making. Examples might relate to such things as student activities, curriculum, or housing regulations. Why is it important for nursing students to concern themselves with these kinds of decisions? Substantiate your answer.

Bibliography

American Nurses' Association (1980). Federation of Specialty Nursing Organizations and ANA: A History. Kansas City, Missouri: The Association.

Bentivegna, G. (1979). Labor Relations: Union Activity Increasing Among Professionals. Hospitals, 53(7):131-140. April 1.

Flanagan, L. (1976). One Strong Voice: The Story of the American Nurses' Association. Kansas City, Missouri: American Nurses' Association.

Gideon, J. (1979). The American Nurses' Association: A Professional Model for Collective Bargaining. Journal of Health and Human Services, 2(1):13-27.

Goode, W. J. (1957). Community Within a Community: The Professions. American Sociological Review, p. 194.

Jacox, A. (1980). Collective Bargaining: The Basis for Professionalism? Supervisor Nurse, 11:22.

Kalisch, B. and Kalisch, P. (1986).The Advance of American Nursing. Boston: Little, Brown and Company.

Lauer, E. F., STD. (1982). Service Strikes: The New Moral Dilemma. In Maida, A. J., editor (1982). Issues in the Labor-Management Dialogue: Church Perspectives. St. Louis: Catholic Health Association of the US.

Levenstein, A. (1980). Professionals and Collective Bargaining. Supervisor Nurse, 11:15.

Merton, R. K. (1958). The Functions of the Professional Association. American Journal of Nursing, 58(1):50.

Muyskens, J. L. (1982). Moral Problems in Nursing: A Philosophical Investigation. Totowa, New Jersey: Rowman and Littlefield.

Muyskens, J. L. (1982). Nurses' Collective Responsibility and the Strike Weapon. Journal of Medicine and Philosophy, 7(1):55.

News (1979). American Journal of Nursing,79(1):7, January.

News (1979). American Journal of Nursing, 79(2):203, February.

News (1979). American Journal of Nursing 79(3):387, March.

O'Rourke, K. A. and Barton, S. R. (1981). Nurse Power: Unions and the Law. Bowie, Maryland: Robert J. Brady Company.

Oppenheimer, M. (1975). The Unionization of the Professional. Social Policy, 5(5):34-40.
Rotkovitch, R. (1980). Do Labor Union Activities Decrease Professionalism? Supervisor Nurse, 11:16.
Shepard, I. M. and Doudera, A., editors (1981). Health Care Labor Law. Ann Arbor, Michigan: AUPHA Press.
Sleicher, M. N. (1981). Nursing Is Not a Profession. Nursing and Health Care, 2(4):186-181.
Wilson, C. N. (1985). Unionization in the Hospital Industry: How Are Wages Affected? Healthcare Financial Management, August, pp. 30-35.

Chapter Ten

THE DEMANDS OF PROFESSION AND THEIR LIMITS

by David Ozar, PhD

The thesis of this book is that being a member of the nursing profession requires a commitment that the individual nurse freely makes to the community at large. This is a commitment not just to think and act wisely, but to do so in accord with the specific values and principles of the nursing profession. This commitment requires careful ethical reflection about clinical ethical issues of nursing practice and about the important professional ethical issues of nursing discussed in the preceding chapters.

Some very important questions still remain, because the ethical demands of professional commitment will not be the only bases of choice and action that a nurse is aware of. Each person knows of other important ethical values and principles besides those implied in the professional commitment. So a tension may well exist between professional principles and other

---

David T. Ozar (PhD, Yale, 1974) is Associate Professor and Director of the Graduate Program in Health Care Ethics, Department of Philosophy, and Adjunct Associate Professor in the Medical Humanities Program, Loyola-Stritch School of Medicine, Loyola University of Chicago. He is also an associate member of the professional staff of Evanston Hospitals, Evanston, Illinois. Dr. Ozar is the author of numerous articles on professional ethics, health care ethics, and social issues. Recently he was the co-editor of *Philosophical Issues in Human Rights: Theories and Applications* (New York: Random House, 1985). He is a frequent lecturer and consultant to professional groups and associations.

principles. We need to ask whether the nurse's professional commitment is a total commitment of the whole person to the values and principles of the profession or a commitment having limits. In order to answer this question, it will be helpful to reflect again on the nature of the nursing profession as a social institution.

Institution, Commitment, and Obligation

Institutions, such as the professions, are for societies what habits are for individual persons. None of us could function very well without our habits, which are patterns of acting in certain ways without further reflection whenever certain sets of circumstances arise. The alternative to habits would be to consciously weigh and judge every possible course of action at every turn of our lives. It is doubtful that we could even get out the door in the morning if we had to judge and choose anew each morning which shoe to put on first or how to hold the toothbrush. In order to make choices thoughtfully about more important matters, we relegate myriad details of our daily lives to habits. We could not function without them.

Institutions function in a similar way within societies. Human interaction depends upon people having a general idea how other people will act or react in numerous situations that people face every day. Numerous social conventions exist in order to provide a stable set of circumstances within which people can attend more carefully to the concerns which are more important to them.

In serving this function, both personal habits and social institutions are inherently conservative. It is their task to preserve unchanged certain patterns of action so there will be a stable framework within which we can make deliberate choices about other matters. Therefore change in habits and institutions requires effort. We can ask ourselves whether a particular habit or institution is somehow getting in the way of the processes of judging and choosing that it is supposed to be assisting, and we can try to change those habits and institutions that are not doing their jobs. Habits are changed by individuals; institutional change requires effort by communities.

One of the chief reasons why the larger community has chosen that nursing be a profession is to *preserve* certain fundamental values and principles in nurses' relationships with other members of the community. Contemporary nursing seems to espouse advocacy, autonomy, and well-being among its fundamental values. The question whether a nurse's professional commitment is to be understood as a *total* commitment of the whole person to these fundamental values and principles, in order to preserve them without qualification, is a very serious one.

To begin to answer it, two distinct sets of norms, or guides for judgment and action, in the nursing profession need examination. One set of these norms is stable; the norms are widely accepted and virtually unchallenged within the profession and in the larger community. The other set of these norms is in flux. They are not universally accepted and are frequently challenged. It may be hard to tell whether they are moving toward greater stability or being increasingly challenged.

At any given time, most of the norms of the nursing profession will be stable. This is what permits us to identify the profession of nursing. But much of the time there will also be some norms of the profession that are in flux. When a particular norm of the profession is in flux, it seems unreasonable to say that a nurse's professional commitment obliges the nurse to respond to it in one way rather than another. If the norm is obviously not derived from one of the fundamental values or principles that define the profession, then each nurse must reflect carefully on the norm in flux and judge what response to it is most in accord with a commitment to the profession's fundamental values and principles. If a firm judgment on this question is possible, then the nurse's professional commitment will have determined, by this reasoning process, how to judge and act about the norm.

If such a judgment is not possible, however, then the nurse might consistently choose either course of action. But having done so, the nurse should then focus on obtaining more understanding of what is at stake in the norm and on more intense dialogue with other nurses and with persons outside the profession regarding the norm, in order to resolve the question of its relation to the fundamental values and principles of nursing.

If the defining fundamental values and principles of the profession are themselves in a state of flux, then the situation is more difficult. If there are competing conceptions of the nature of nursing so radically different that the nurse's daily practice would be significantly changed by a shift from one conception to the other, then there is not even a significant continuity of daily practice to carry the members of the profession along while they and the larger community work out their fundamental uncertainties about the nature of the profession. For a profession does not simply define itself, but works out its character and definition in dialogue with the larger community (Ozar, 1985). On the other hand, if the rival understandings of the profession imply similar norms for much of daily practice, then at least these norms can be acted on by all, even as the fundamental issues are debated and worked out.

But what of the stable norms of the profession? Must a nurse's commitment to these norms be total and unqualified or are there limits to the obligations that these norms imply? To answer these questions, we need to examine three bases of an obligation to adhere to the stable norms of a profession: (1) the professional's act of commitment, (2) the value of stability, and (3) the underlying values and principles which the profession serves within the community.

Commitment

One reason why a professional is obligated to judge and act in certain ways is that he or she has made a *commitment* to do so. The act of commitment is like making a promise or making a contract. In all of these acts, a person voluntarily undertakes to be obligated to act (or refrain from acting) in certain ways for the benefit of another person or group of persons.

The act of professional commitment is unlike making a promise and making a contract, however, because of the particular character of the professional-client relationship, which varies from profession to profession. As explained in an earlier chapter, the client of the health professional is at once autonomous and dependent, in specific ways, and is therefore significantly different from both the receiver of a promise and the co-maker of a contract (Ozar, 1984; Veatch, 1981).

When we say that one source of a professional's obligations is the professional's own undertaking of these obligations, we mean that acting contrary to the norms of the profession after the commitment has been made contradicts one's own choice. It violates a person's consistency, integrity, and wholeness as a person. We shall return to these themes of commitment and wholeness as a person in the next section. First, we need to inquire whether an act of professional commitment, and the obligations to which it gives rise, are necessarily unconditional, and in that sense constitute a total commitment of one's whole person.

In most acts of promising, and in many contractual situations as well, important elements of the promise or contract are not stated explicitly. They are implicit at the time the promise or contract is made, and are made explicit only later if the need to state them arises. If I make a promise to visit my ailing uncle in the nursing home, but I don't show up because my child has become ill and I have taken her to the doctor, few people would claim that I have broken my promise. There are implicit conditions on such promises, conditions concerning personal and familial emergencies, which are rarely stated or even attended to when the promise is made, but which everyone can understand as being implicit elements of such promises from the start.

In a similar way, there is much about a professional commitment that is implicit. The formal declaration of commitment that is publicly spoken and the profession's published code of ethics are often the only fully explicit elements of a professional commitment. They cannot address all the activities of a profession's practice. It is taken for granted that there is much that is unsaid but understood from the start.

There are several ways in which implicit conditions on the professional's commitment will appear to limit the professional's obligations. First, the professional is surely committed above all to the fundamental values and principles that define the profession. These values or principles will guide the professional's judgment and action even when they conflict with public declarations of commitment or the profession's formal code of ethics. The professional may be placed at some risk in such a situation because the required action may appear to directly violate the profession's norms. But in the best of situations the professional's explanation of the action, showing that it conforms to the fundamental values and principles of the profession, will suffice. In the case discussed in Chapter 6, for example, Joleen Tuma appeared to believe that in violating a professional norm she was being true to her professional commitment.

Second, there may be other kinds of limitations implicit in professional commitment. Is a nurse's professional obligation limited by personal or familial emergencies? Would failure to perform professional duties (for example, to distribute medications or to instruct a patient being discharged regarding proper diet) still be unprofessional conduct if the reason were a personal or familial emergency?

A first answer to these questions would probably be that the nurse should find another nurse to take over these tasks. This would fulfill the nurse's professional obligations under the circumstances. But suppose a nurse did not do this either, because of the same personal or familial emergency? I believe such an act would be unprofessional, a violation of the nurse's professional commitment to judge and act in certain ways. If my judgment is correct here, then the nurse's professional commitment is not limited by this particular implicit condition. Acts that are unprofessional might still be ethically justified, however, if they are based on other important values and principles besides those of the profession. That question will be examined in the next section.

Stability

A second reason why a professional is obligated to judge and act in certain ways is the value of stability within important human relationships. As already indicated, the nursing profession is a social institution that exists because of its acceptance and support by the larger community. One reason why the community accepts and supports this institution is the community's need for stability and dependability in relationships between those who need health care and those who provide it. If a nurse violates professional commitments, her actions undermine this important community value. Again, we must ask if adherence to this value must be unconditional. There are three distinct beneficiaries of a nurse's stable performance of professional obligations: the community at large, other members of the nursing profession, and each individual nurse. We will look at these in turn.

Patients, prospective patients, and those who are relatives and friends of patients constitute the community at large. All of them value a stable set of relationships between nurses and patients and between nurses and other participants in the health care system. They want these to be stable relationships so they can concentrate their attention on the difficult tasks of dealing with illness, cooperating with therapy, and returning to their normal lives. Interruptions of the patterns of these relationships are experienced as disturbing, sometimes profoundly so.

Yet it might not be stability itself that is valued in these relationships, but rather the stable and assured impact of those values and principles that make the nurse-patient relationship as beneficial as possible to the patient and, secondarily, to those who love and support the patient. Ideally the values and principles that define the nursing profession are the fruit of a dialogue between the profession and the larger community. This dialogue is aimed precisely at shaping the best possible nurse-patient relationship. Professional obligation gives priority to the fundamental values and principles of nursing even if they conflict with a particular accepted practice. Thus stability is an *instrumental* value. It gains its worth from what it leads to, i.e., the most beneficial nurse-patient relationship possible. It is therefore a limited value, to be sacrificed when that relationship will be better without it. So the obligations of nurses to which the value of stability gives rise are also limited by the fundamental values and principles of nursing which that value serves.

Stability is also a value to the members of the profession because it enables them to know what to expect from each other. Without such stability in the meeting of professional obligations, nurses would find it extremely difficult to coordinate their work, both in the sense of working together at common tasks and in the sense of following one another sequentially at the same tasks, as shift follows shift within health care institutions. Other issues beyond the performance of individual tasks also demand stable values in the profession. Standards for education and licensing, for example, require a shared, stable conception of the profession and its commitment. The purpose of such coordination of effort is to provide the best possible nursing care for patients and appropriate assistance for those who love and support them. So once again stability is a limited, instrumental value in the service of the fundamental values and principles of nursing.

Finally, stability in the profession's performance of its obligations is a value to each individual nurse in several ways. It can provide emotional support and reinforce individual efforts to make the fundamental values and principles of nursing into personal habits of judgment and action. It can provide insight into how to apply these values and principles in the daily activities of nursing practice. It can also simplify the process of judgment in difficult cases by providing the nurse with the stable practice of the profession as evidence in support of one course of action over another. Once again stability of practice serves as an instrumental value, enhancing each nurse's ability to apply nursing's fundamental values and principles in practice.

But there is a danger here as well. It is possible for stability in others' practice to become a crutch, replacing concrete judgments by the individual nurse. Stability can seem to relieve the nurse of the burden of judgment in matters that ought to be thought out and decided on the basis of clinical and nonclinical facts and relevant ethical and professional values rather than on the basis of some pattern observed in others and borrowed for the purpose. Obviously when the concern for stability in the patterns of nursing practice has led a nurse to refrain from personal professional judgment, it has gone beyond its bounds.

The Fundamental Values and Principles of Nursing

The most important basis of a nurse's obligation to judge and act in certain ways is the fundamental values and principles that define the nursing profession and that are embodied concretely in the nurse-patient relationship. The foregoing examinations of commitment and of the value of stability have served only to reinforce and clarify the primacy of these fundamental values and principles as the basis of nurses' professional obligation. But again we must ask if such professional obligation, grounded in these values and principles, is absolute, total, unlimited.

To answer this question we must ask another question, which was introduced in passing a few pages back. Can actions by nurses that deliberately violate the fundamental values and principles of nursing, and thus clearly violate professional commmitment, nevertheless be ethical if they are based on a person's other important ethical values and principles? Answering this question will require us to return to the theme of the act of commitment and to focus our attention on commitment as the act of a nurse as a whole person.

THE NURSE AS A WHOLE PERSON

Professional Values and the "Minimum" Test

Under some conditions it is certainly ethical for a nurse to knowingly choose to act in violation of professional obligation. A nurse, after careful and conscientious consideration of the alternative actions available, might sincerely judge that the morally required course of action in some situations is not the course of action required by the nurse's professional commitment. It should not be news that a person ought to do what, after careful and conscientious reflection, he or she sincerely judges to be ethically required in the situation. This does not limit professional or any other kind of obligation, but rather states the meaning of responsibility for acting ethically in the first place.

Almost all of us first learned ethical behavior by doing as we were told because certain others were better judges of morality than we were or because certain systems of rules were better guides to ethical action than our own judgments were. This was very likely the case when we were children, but one mark of growth into adulthood is increasing ability to understand for ourselves the ethical significance of our actions, to reflect carefully and conscientiously on our alternatives, and to judge wisely how to act. This does not mean that we can learn nothing from others or that various systems of rules have nothing to teach us. It means that our acceptance of guidance from either of these sources is itself an act of judgment and choice that we must make for ourselves, thoughtfully and wisely.

Therefore to say that people ought to act as they carefully and conscientiously judge they ought to act, even if this means violating professional obligations, does not place a limit on professional commitment. It states an inherent feature of human moral responsibility. Instead the question that must concern us is whether there is something about an act of professional commitment such that no other moral considerations could possibly outweigh or overrule the obligations that this commitment implies.

In order to understand this question, we need to remember that most people value many different kinds of things and are members of many different kinds of communities, playing many different roles in them and having the capacity to live a part of their lives independently of any roles at all. (By a "role" I mean a set of relationships and tasks, and a set of values and principles of conduct to define them, that are accepted and thereby established as having a certain normative function within a given community.) If this were not true, there would be no tension between the obligations implied by a person's professional commitment and either the other values and principles that the person esteems or the other roles, with their implied obligations, to which the person has made commitment. Most professionals experience such tension; the question is whether this tension must always be resolved in the same way. Must a conscientious, carefully thinking person who has made a professional commitment always judge thereafter that, for him or her, professional obligation must override all other ethical considerations?

If the commitment is something real, then it must make a difference. One might think that this implies that professional obligation must win out whenever there is a conflict of obligations. But I believe that commitment to a set of fundamental values and principles can make a difference without it being the case that these values and principles must invariably overrule all other ethical considerations. I shall now try to show this.

In order to outline an alternative description of professional commitment, I shall propose that we humans can learn to recognize very subtle discriminations in comparing and ranking specific ethical values and principles. We do not always do this perfectly, but we do have the ability to make such discriminations in most of the situations in which we need to make ethical judgments. When we single out a particular value or principle or set of them for special attention, we are not limited to saying only, "It will always win," or "It will never win." We can also say something like this: "It will overrule values and principles of one sort, but it will not overrule values and principles of another sort."

The professional's commitment is, I propose, of the latter sort. It is not a commitment to invariably weigh the fundamental values and principles of one's profession above all other possible ethical considerations. It is instead a commitment to rank these professional values in such a way that only ethical considerations of a specified minimum degree of importance can ever outweigh them. This minimum is part of the definition of each profession, but the content of this "minimum" for each profession is best learned from the actual patterns of practice of the profession. A few brief illustrations of this "minimum" for nursing can be offered here.

The commitment to nursing is a commitment to value the well-being of the nurse's patients more than the well-being of any other persons, including self. Only the risk of immediate loss of life (or something sincerely judged to be of comparable value and importance) on the part of a nonpatient can equal or outweigh the well-being of a nurse's patient, and then only if the service of this other person does not place the patient's life in comparable risk. Nothing of lesser value or importance can outweigh a nurse's meeting the nursing needs of the patient in an appropriate and timely fashion. (This statement is still too general, because nursing practice involves numerous concrete judgments regarding patient need, the timing of needed care, and the distribution of the nurse's limited time on duty. Therefore, implicit in the "minimum" are numerous features of concrete nursing practice that cannot be explained without detailed study of cases from actual practice.)

A nurse is also committed to valuing the patient's autonomy so highly that, even if the nurse sincerely judges that a patient is choosing a worse path rather than a better one but is doing so with full capacity for judgment and choice and with full understanding of the relevant facts, then the nurse will not interfere with the carrying out of the patient's choice and will work for the patient's maximum well-being in the context of that choice. Here the "minimum" is defined in terms of the patient's capacity to understand, judge, and choose. Only if there is good reason to doubt the patient's capacity will the value of the patient's well-being as conceived by the nurse, or the health care team or institution, be ranked above the patient's own conception of well-being and the patient's own choices.

Also, the nurse is committed to serving as advocate in the patient's dependency, both the dependency of injury or illness and the dependency of position within the health care system. This means that the nurse will work to enhance the patient's capacity for choice and to prevent the patient from being relegated by institutional roles, relationships, or routine into an unnecessarily passive and dependent position. The "minimum" here is difficult to describe. Perhaps the nurse is committed to ranking the patient's need for advocacy above all bureaucratic and role-related obstacles short of those that would make the nurse ineffective as the patient's advocate in the first place. For example, if advocacy for a particular patient on some matter would, if carried further, bring about the nurse's transfer by higher authority to another unit or the nurse's dismissal from employment, then the nurse's professional commitment to advocacy would not ordinarily require the nurse to take any further steps. The reason would be that, if transferred or dismissed, the nurse can no longer serve effectively as the patient's advocate in any case. This is the sort of "minimum" test that values other than advocacy would have to meet before they could be judged to equal or outweigh it. (This example has focused on advocacy for a single patient in some specific matter. If the patient's case is representative of a larger, systematic inadequacy in the roles, relationships, or bureaucracy of the institution, the nurse's commitment to advocacy may require or at least justify actions beyond the "minimum" just described, as acts aimed at changing the system for all the nurse's patients, present and future.)

Thus the nurse's commitment, I am proposing, does not exclude values and principles other than those of nursing itself from being taken into account in the nurse's judgments, choices, and actions. It is a commitment, instead, that the values and principles of nursing will have a high and fixed level of importance in the nurse's life. Other values and principles will be able to equal or outweigh them only in circumstances in which they pass a very high "minimum" test of importance themselves. In this respect the nurse's commitment is a limited and not a total one though it is clearly very significant.

The Nurse on Duty

This description of the nurse's commitment might appear to be asking too much, however, even though it speaks of limits, until we consider the crucial concept of being *on duty*. The commitment just described applies with full force only during the time that a nurse is *on duty* and only in regard to those patients for whom the nurse is considered responsible while on duty, the patients *in the nurse's care*.

By "time on duty" I mean not only the actual period of paid employment but also, depending on the circumstances, periods of time before or after the period of paid employment, and possibly at other times as well. Thus the nurse's commitment may require coming in a few minutes early or staying late for the sake of a particular patient or a group of patients in the unit. These times are part of a nurse's time *on duty*. Several other examples of such extensions of time *on duty* will be discussed later. The point is that the nurse's time on duty is finite, rarely extending beyond, say, 50 hours per week. During the rest of the nurse's life, the professional commitment does not oblige in the same way as has been described.

By "patients in the nurse's care" I mean primarily the patients for whom the nurse has primary responsibility within the nurse's home unit. Obviously a nurse also has responsibility for the care of all the patients on the unit if need should arise and for other patients within that institution as well, depending on the circumstances. If a nurse were on break, for example, and an ambulating patient from another unit collapsed nearby while the nurse was walking to the cafeteria, the nurse would be responsible to care for that patient until others who have responsibility for the patient were available. But if a nurse observed an auto accident from a patient's window, even if it looked like it involved serious injuries, the nurse's professional responsibilities would be to the patients on the unit rather than the victims of the accident. This means that the nurse's professional commitment, while requiring a high degree of altruism, does not require a nurse to act altruistically toward every person in the nurse's life. The extent of obligations implied by the nursing commitment during times when a nurse is off duty and toward persons not in the nurse's care are a matter of some dispute. Both of these topics will be addressed in a later section of this chapter, "Changing Fallible Institutions."

With these things said, we can return to the theme of the nurse as a whole person. Like any human being, a nurse values many different kinds of things and is a member of many different communities, playing many different roles and living part of life (or at least able to live part of life) independently of any roles. When a nurse is on duty, the other values, commitments, and communities of a nurse's life must, for the most part (except as determined by the "minimum" tests explained earlier), play a secondary role. But in the rest of the nurse's life, they will rightly play whatever role the nurse judges and chooses they should play.

Some people live psychologically sound and happy lives devoted almost exclusively to the values and relationships of a single profession. But for most people a broader range of values and relationships is esteemed, and participation in a broader range of communities and in a broader range of roles is needed for happiness and psychological health. Most people make a commitment to another person as husband or wife. Most establish lasting friendships with other adults. Most make the commitment of parenthood to children and the commitments of adult children to parents, commitments to other family members, and so on. All of these relationships and numerous other values are part of the ordinary life of most nurses.

There is no conflict between such values and nursing. There is no reason to say that the values and principles of nursing should somehow dominate all the rest of a nurse's life. The nurse's commitment is to the *dominance* of these values and principles (qualified by the "minimum" tests indicated earlier) only when the nurse is *on duty* and only toward those patients *in the nurse's care*. Such a commitment requires significant sacrifice and an admirable degree of altruism under often trying circumstances. It sometimes pushes the best of us to our limits. Yet it is not an absolute commitment, without limits or qualifications, nor a total resignation of one's whole life and every shred of one's self to the values and principles of nursing. It is, or can be in a balanced and thoughtful person, a rich and demanding but also a balanced and possible commitment, the commitment of a whole, multivalued person.

PROBLEMS AND TENSION

A careful account of the fundamental values and principles of nursing and of the most important bases of ethical thinking does not constitute a black box into which someone can feed data about a particular situation and turn the crank to get the answer about what a nurse ought or ought not do. Neither is an account of the limits of professional commitment (like this chapter) a source of easy answers to subtle questions about ethical action. Many problems and tensions remain. I shall briefly examine here several of these problems and tensions in order to explain how some of what has been said in this chapter might be applied concretely.

Disaffection with Nursing

It is a long-standing principle of ethical reflection that we are never obligated to do what is truly impossible. When people make commitments, they commit themselves to maintain at a certain high level of importance a particular value or principle or set of values and principles and to act accordingly in all ways within their power. Thus if nurses feel a spontaneous aversion toward a particular patient, they are obligated to do what they can to "set that feeling aside" and provide that patient the same measure of care as any other. Most often such challenges are manageable, and when the strain involved is excessive or may compromise patient care, a nurse is usually able to find a way for another member of the staff to take primary responsibility for that patient. We do not consider such feelings to be violations of professional nursing because we recognize that, while we can ordinarily control what we *do*, we cannot always control our *feelings*, including feelings regarding particular persons.

But what if a nurse feels disaffection for the practice of nursing itself? It would be a natural reaction to judge oneself very harshly for feelings of disaffection towards one's profession, as if all such feelings could be controlled. While some of our feelings can be controlled or moderated by reflecting on them or discussing them with others or through changes in other aspects of our lives, other feelings do not respond to such efforts.

Most people experience times when they feel tired of or angry at all the day-in, day-out sacrifices and frustrations of their professional lives. Having such feelings is not a violation of one's professional commitment. Instead, the relevant question is what we *do*, how we act when we experience such feelings.

Sometimes, for some people, feelings of disaffection with the nurse's role establish themselves as a constant pattern in their lives. Such feelings may be impervious to thoughtful reflection or dialogue or to other efforts to moderate or change them. They may persist and may concern the most fundamental aspects of the nurse-patient relationship. Here again there may well be no violation of professional commitment in the existence of such feelings. Their strength may be beyond a person's control, or be the consequence of perfectly legitimate and ethical changes in other aspects of a person's life. But continuance in a way of life ordinarily depends upon a person's having supportive or at least neutral feelings regarding it. Therefore a persistent and substantive disaffection with nursing may indicate the wisdom of choosing to withdraw from the profession, at least temporarily. Though painful for a person sincerely committed to the service of others, such a choice need not violate professional commitment. There are many ways of serving others *and* achieving our own happiness. Professionals have not committed themselves to the impossible.

Joining a Fallible Profession

One of the most important themes of this book is that those who intend to enter the nursing profession should study and understand the commitment they propose to make. It is by making this commitment that a person becomes a nurse. But the content of this commitment, the values and principles that define the nursing profession and the roles and relationships that embody them, is the work of the whole profession and the larger community working together in dialogue. It is not created there and then by the one who makes the commitment.

Thus there is a sense in which the prospective nurse must "take it or leave it," and this may be a source of tension or uncertainty about commitment to the profession when the profession that one must "take or leave" is a fallible human institution. Is one's commitment a commitment to this profession *as it is*, warts and all? Or is it a commitment to the profession's *ideals*, to which it aspires but which it only partially achieves at any given time? How are we to understand this commitment?

Each prospective nurse will need to formulate a personal answer to these questions after reflecting carefully on the actual character of the profession. Is it significantly flawed? Is it fallible but struggling to improve? Is it fairly successful in living up to its ideals? Is it almost without stain or wrinkle? In each case, a person can still make a commitment to the fundamental values and principles of nursing while working for a higher degree, or a continued high degree, of fulfillment of these ideals in the profession. The difference will be in differing degrees of loyalty to the profession as it is and to the profession as it ought to be. Each of these responses is consistent with an act of commitment to the profession.

What is not consistent with professional commitment is serious doubt about and withholding one's commitment from the fundamental values and principles of the profession. It is with regard to these that the prospective nurse must "take it or leave it." A particular individual who had such doubts or reservations might still go through all the steps of admission to the profession and then appear to all the world to be committed to the profession's values and principles, while nevertheless intending to work from the "inside" to change those values and principles to better ones. Though this path might be chosen on the basis of thoughtful ethical reflection on the kinds of institutions best suited to achieve human well-being, the position of such a person is still an anomaly. It is hard to describe such a person as a full member, or a fully committed member, of the profession. For again the fundamental values and principles that define the nursing profession are not created by the individual nurse who makes a commitment to them; they are the work of all the members of the profession and the larger community, working together in dialogue.

The same things can also be said of an experienced member of the profession. Every nurse should stop and reflect regularly on the extent to which the nursing profession, in its individual members and as a group, is living up to the values and principles that define it and to the ideal fulfillment of the values and principles to which it aspires. When weaknesses are found, the nurse's commitment to these values and principles in the profession requires effort to improve it.

All nurses should also periodically examine their own personal commitment to these professional values and principles. If there is now serious doubt about them or a genuine withdrawing of commitment, it may be best for such a person to withdraw from the profession, unless alternative values and principles for the profession are seen and the person chooses the anomalous position just described from which to work to change the profession in the direction of these other values and principles.

Changing Fallible Institutions

The extent to which a nurse's professional commitment implies an obligation to support the work of the profession within the larger society has been discussed in Chapter 9. But nurses deal with many other institutions besides their own profession and the larger society. They deal with hospitals and their administrations and with other departments and service units, with other professional groups, and with many other institutions structured economically, politically, socially, culturally. In some cases nurses are members of the institutions with which they deal; in others they are outsiders. All of these are fallible human institutions, and a nurse will often experience the consequences of their fallibility. When the flaws of such institutions compromise nurses' ability to care for patients in accord with the fundamental values and principles of nursing, do nurses then have a professional obligation to work to change these institutions?

One possible answer to this question would limit the nurse's obligation by reminding us that a person is committed to judging and acting according to the values and principles of her or his profession only in matters within the person's own control. There is no obligation to do what is not possible. Therefore, it might be argued, if surrounding institutions set limits on a nurse's ability to fulfill professional obligations in the most ideal fashion, then the nurse is truly obligated only to do the best possible within these limits.

But this answer overlooks the fact that, besides being fallible, human institutions are also changeable. The limits they place on the provision of the best nursing care are not necessarily absolute. The nurse's obligation to fulfill the values and principles of nursing requires at a minimum a thoughtful examination of the institutions at fault, a reflection on possible alternatives that would be less compromising of proper nursing care, and a look at possible strategies for the achievement of these alternatives. The result of such deliberation may be a judgment that the relevant institutions are immovable, at least practically speaking. But more often than not such deliberation will reveal avenues of recourse for those who are willing to participate in the process of dialogue by which new institutions are created and existing institutions changed.

Reflection on strategies for change may also indicate that the impetus for dialogue will depend upon more voices than that of a single nurse. Failed efforts to achieve dialogue with the involved parties or the failure of dialogue to initiate needed changes may indicate that change will not occur without the addition of many voices to the process. It seems obvious that a nurse would be obligated to at least initiate dialogue toward institutional change when the proper achievement of the fundamental values and principles of nursing is at stake. But when sound strategies for change require that many voices be raised together, the situation becomes complicated by the interplay of many values. Careful judgments of the relative merits of several different courses of action will have to be made. The extent to which fundamental values and principles of nursing are truly at stake, the relative importance of other values and principles that are involved, and the "minimum" implicit in nursing's professional commitment—all of these will need to be weighed for a careful judgment and choice of appropriate action.

As soon as the impetus for change requires many voices to be effective, we are necessarily talking about *political* action. Beyond simply communicating to others about an ongoing dialogue, we must begin to talk about mustering support, selecting leaders and spokespersons, and identifying other persons or groups as being, at least in this matter, the "opposition." Those espousing some views of nursing argue that nurses *must* engage in such political activities when the fundamental values and principles of nursing are truly compromised by institutions in need of change. If political action is the only means available for effecting the needed change, they argue, then nurses are professionally obligated to participate. Those with other views of nursing would hold that such activities are profoundly inimical to the values and principles of nursing and therefore violate a nurse's professional commitment.

The focus on the notion of "time on duty," developed earlier, might seem to automatically lift the burden of political activism from the nurse's shoulders in another way. The nurse's commitment, it was proposed, applies with full force only during the time that a nurse is *on duty* and only to those patients who are in the nurse's care. So, it might be argued, a nurse is not obligated to participate in political activity to change institutions when the nurse is off duty, and surely it is a rare nurse who would have time while on duty to engage in significant political activity. Therefore, it might be concluded, a nurse's professional obligation to participate in such activity is minimal.

It is important to remember, however, that the notion of "time on duty" is not limited to the actual period of paid employment. It also includes such other periods of time, most often (but not necessarily) immediately before or after the period of paid employment, as are crucial for the proper care of the nurse's patients. A nurse could conceivably be professionally obligated to pick up a patient's records or lab reports or visit a patient's family during unpaid time, depending on the details of the particular care. Because of the patient's situation, this would be genuine time *on duty*, even if unpaid. Similarly, a nurse might be professionally obligated to try to change flawed institutional structures that were compromising a patient's care. If it were the only available way to do this, a nurse might be obligated to participate in appropriate political action to achieve it. If so, this too would be part of the nurse's time *on duty,* as this concept is being used here. Therefore a nurse's professional commitment does not rule out political action, nor does it always require it. The specific circumstances of the situation will determine whether this is an appropriate or necessary means for providing proper care to the nurse's patients.

Political action can take many forms. Organization, dissemination of information, lobbying, public meetings and demonstrations, legal action, and use of the print and broadcast media can all be part of this process. So too can acts of institutional "civil disobedience," i.e., the deliberate and public violation of an institutional rule, judged to be harmful or unethical, for the explicit purpose of bringing about dialogue or political action to change it, and with the known risk of suffering institutional penalties for the violation. So too are boycotts and strikes, which have already been discussed in Chapter 9. In all these activities both individual participants and groups working together must carefully examine the other outcomes of such activities, over and above their effectiveness in furthering the cause. If the activities are producing or might produce unintended harm, either to participants or especially to noninvolved third parties who might otherwise be overlooked, the activities must be subjected to very careful ethical examination before being undertaken or continued.

The Nurse Off Duty

To what extent does a nurse's professional commitment touch the rest of the nurse's life? Let us consider the view that the commitment to the fundamental values and principles of nursing must be evident in every judgment and choice of a nurse's life, that the nurse must be a living symbol and exemplar of these values and principles to the community. Thus, for example, nurses who smoke or are significantly overweight by reason of eating habits or lifestyle would be violating the nurse's professional commitment to place a very high value on people's well-being and its physiological foundations by not embodying these in their daily lives.

A point made earlier would seem to contradict this view. Does it not follow from what has already been said that what a nurse does when not on duty is the nurse's own business and has no relation to the nurse's professional commitment? In reflecting on this argument we must first recall that a nurse's time on duty often includes other times and activities besides those that make up the nurse's paid employment because the obligation to the nurse's patients may extend beyond the hours on a time card. But, having said this, it may still be proper for us to stress the limits of a nurse's professional obligation; for a nurse's professional commitment implies obligations only toward the patients in the nurse's care. From this it would follow that a nurse is not professionally obligated to represent or symbolize the values and principles of nursing to the community at large and therefore is not *professionally* obligated to attend to her or his own well-being, for example, except insofar as it is related to providing appropriate nursing care to the nurse's own patients.

This surely means that nurses are obligated to care for their own health in ways that would directly affect patient care when they are on duty. So drug and alcohol dependency, whose effects on judgment and performance cannot be limited to the hours a nurse is off duty, clearly violate a nurse's professional commitment. Similarly, if substitute caregivers were really in such short supply in a particular institution that a nurse's absence because of illness would seriously compromise patient care, then the nurse might well be professionally obligated to take more than ordinary care of personal health for the sake of patients. But in less extreme situations, a nurse's professional obligation to care for patients requires only ordinary care of the nurse's own personal health.

In a similar way, it would be psychologically difficult for a nurse on duty to care for patients as an advocate and in a manner deeply affirmative of their autonomy if the nurse's life off duty were one of habitual manipulation of and dominance over others. Habitual patterns of thought and relationship affect all our judgments and actions. Moreover, most people experience the need to live by a fairly unified and coherent set of values and principles. This means that an off-duty life lived in profound conflict with the fundamental values and principles of nursing will create great tensions in a nurse's life on duty, and very likely will lead to serious disaffection for nursing. So a choice to habitually follow such a path in the rest of one's life will almost always be inconsistent with a professional commitment to nursing.

Yet we have still not resolved the larger question of whether the nurse is professionally committed to being a symbol or exemplar to the larger community. It is certainly conceivable that a profession could do so. So it is not an absurdity to think of a profession undertaking this task. The question is whether the nursing profession has undertaken it, and done so in such a way that it is a part of the commitment that every nurse makes. This question can be answered only by consulting the current state of the dialogue between the nursing profession and the larger community about the nature of the nursing profession. The larger community does not presently seem to be asking or expecting nurses to be role models of certain values or principles. The community at large seems to believe that the nurse is not professionally obligated in any particular way, except possibly in emergency situations, which we will examine shortly. If this is in fact how the community, in dialogue with the nursing profession, understands the nurse's professional commitment, then this is how it is.

Of course, individual institutions within the larger community may choose to follow more restrictive paths. For example, Westlake Community Hospital in the Chicago suburb of Melrose Park, Illinois, recently instituted an employment policy requiring new workers to be nonsmokers, even away from work ("Smokers Fuming Over Ban," *Chicago Sun Times,* February 3, 1985, p. 16). A nurse's obligations with regard to institutional actions of this sort will depend upon the nature of the nurse's commitment, if any, to the institution itself and on the other values and principles of conduct that the nurse esteems, as well as the values and principles of nursing. The nurse's professional commitment does not point to clear obligations either way on such matters.

One possible exception to this account of a nurse's professional obligations when off duty is the "Good Samaritan" situation, in which someone who is not a patient in a nurse's care experiences a health emergency in the presence of the nurse. Suppose a nurse is riding a bus when one of the passengers gets ill. Is the nurse professionally obligated to come to the sick person's aid? Does it matter if the nurse is wearing an identifying uniform or is known to someone present as being a nurse? What does the nurse's professional commitment require in such a situation?

There is considerable ambiguity about the community's expectations of nurses in situations of this sort; therefore necessarily some doubt exists about the content of the nurse's professional commitment regarding them. Almost certainly a nurse would be obligated to offer whatever assistance possible to a person whose life was clearly or even only probably at risk, either because of illness or serious injury.

Although this is an ethical obligation, it is not clear that it is a *professional* obligation. For anyone, regardless of expertise or commitment, would seem to be obligated in almost any theory of ethics to assist a person who was probably at risk of death or serious injury, up to the limit of their ability to help without comparable risk to themselves. The difference with the nurse, then, may not be that the nurse has a specific professional obligation to assist but rather that the nurse has the same obligation that any adult would have, and has much more to offer.

If this is so, then the nurse's obligation to assist persons in lesser need could be outweighed by other values and principles esteemed by the nurse, just as anyone's obligation to assist could be outweighed in the same situation. Suppose, for example, that the person in need did not appear to be seriously ill or in any significant risk of more serious complications and was already receiving the common sense attention of other persons nearby. There would not seem to be any professional obligation on the nurse's part to assist in this sort of situation. Of course a nurse might respond more readily than others simply because the nurse actually values ministering to others' health care needs more than most members of the community. But this does not mean that the nurse has a special *professional* obligation to assist. The nurse's obligation would be the same obligation that we all have to help persons in need, depending upon the seriousness of their need and our particular abilities.

If a nurse happens, for some reason, to be known or recognized by those present in such a situation, the nurse will then have a special reason besides the reasons just mentioned for offering assistance. It is an important feature of the relationship between the nursing profession and the larger community that the latter be assured that nurses assign a very high value to others' well-being, especially in relation to their health. Though the nurse might otherwise have no obligation to rank another's well-being over the other values and principles which that particular nurse esteems, this additional factor of supporting, rather than challenging, the community's (correct) convictions regarding the nursing profession will frequently weigh the scales in the direction of offering assistance. But such professional obligation as there is in such a situation is in the form of an obligation to the *profession* to work for its well-being, not an obligation to the person in (less than serious) need.

Because the focus of a nurse's professional commitment is on the proper care of those patients for whom the nurse is responsible, the focus of this commitment is on the "time on duty," when the nurse is directly or indirectly ministering to them. In the rest of a nurse's life and in the nurse's dealings with other persons, the professional commitment of the nurse, as it currently exists, implies few obligations. Instead, all of a nurse's values and principles of conduct, which include but are not limited to the values and principles of nursing, must be considered thoughtfully together in judging which actions are ethical and best, and which are not.

Conscientious Refusal

An examination of one final, special situation will complete this chapter. This is the situation in which there is a profound conflict between what a nurse's personal morality, formed in careful and conscientious reflection on what is most important in human life, requires in a situation and what the nurse's professional obligations are in the situation. The most frequently discussed example of such conflicts at the present time concerns nurses' participation in abortion procedures. The nurse's professional duty is to the patient, not only to serve the patient's health but to respect the patient's autonomy and serve as an advocate for the patient within the health care system. But what if the nurse has formed, after careful consideration of the matter, a sincere judgment not only that certain (or all) abortions are immoral for those women who seek them and also that it is immoral for a nurse to participate in certain (or all) abortion procedures? What is the ethical thing for a nursing professional to do under such circumstances?

In many institutions it is possible for a nurse who would be faced with a profound ethical conflict if assigned to assist in abortion procedures simply to arrange for assignment elsewhere. It will often be possible for a nurse to arrange for other nurses to assist in such a procedure if the situation arises in a unit in which it is otherwise unlikely. In such situations, the ethical challenge for the nurse is more often that of deciding whether to be employed by, and thus lend indirect or symbolic support to, an institution that performs abortions, which the nurse judges to be immoral. While this may indeed be a difficult ethical decision, a nurse would rarely if ever have a professional obligation to work at a particular health care institution. Nor does a nurse have a professional obligation to practice in any particular area of health care. Consequently a nurse's specifically professional obligations may not be involved in such decisions.

But suppose a situation arises in which a nurse cannot avoid choosing between neglecting a particular patient in need and assisting in a procedure that the nurse judges to be immoral. Can or should a nurse's professional obligation to attend to the patient's well-being outweigh the nurse's deepest, most conscientiously held values and principles? The proposal I wish to make is that we *cannot* commit ourselves to set aside our most deeply held ethical values and principles. They are the basis of our choices to make important commitments, including professional commitments, in the first place. We do not make commitments, particularly commitments involving serious, long-term obligations, out of thin air, for no particular reason at all. Most often we make them, if we make them seriously, for the deepest and most important of our reasons for doing anything. It is therefore inconsistent, I propose, to say that there are commitments that may not ethically be violated no matter what is at stake.

The crucial question for the decision-maker in a situation of profound ethical conflict, then, is to try to determine which of the relevant values and principles are indeed the most basic, and then whether they are basic enough that they must take precedence over the obligations implied by professional commitment. When such is the case, we can call the act an act of "conscientious refusal" (Rawls, 1971, pp. 268-371). It is an instance, perhaps the most striking instance, in which a person ought to do what he or she sincerely and conscientiously judges ought to be done, which is precisely what we are speaking of when we describe ourselves as morally responsible beings.

The challenge of such situations is to know our deepest values and convictions well enough to make such judgments wisely. Self-knowledge does not come to us on the spur of the moment; it requires thoughtful reflection and, for most of us, thoughtful, honest, respectful dialogue with other concerned persons about what really is most important in human life and what our professional commitments are really about. Such reflection and dialogue are not easy and are not common. But our ability to respond properly and wisely in situations of profound ethical conflict depends upon our fostering them in our own lives and for others.

SUMMARY

In this chapter, David Ozar has carefully distinguished an individual's professional commitment from other sets of values and principles which govern that person's actions. It is appropriate that his comments should conclude this volume, because they provide a framework within which to balance the professional commitment with the rest of one's life. In previous chapters we have emphasized the individual and collective responsibilities that individuals accept when they choose to enter the profession of nursing. Ozar points out that although the commitment to a profession is serious, fulfilling that commitment should not require one to violate another, more fundamental personal ethic. Ozar provides some concrete examples of the tensions between values that nurses commonly encounter and suggests how they can be analyzed. He challenges readers to know their own deepest values and convictions well enough that when conflicts arise, they can make a morally responsible decision, even if that decision means refusing to participate in a professionally required activity.

For Further Discussion

1. Review Ozar's discussion of "the nurse on duty" and the explanation that the primary commitment of nursing applies with full force only during the time that a nurse is on duty and only in regard to those patients for whose care the nurse is considered responsible while on duty. Discuss how the practice environment and the roles in which a nurse functions might affect the ease with which this concept could be utilized. How would this argument apply when the nurse is functioning as a primary nurse? A community health nurse? A nurse midwife?

2. Chapter 4 presented the case of Nurse Munson and Mrs. Brumley, the terminally ill patient whose physician provided a PRN order for an unusually large dose of pain medication. Consider this situation within the context of Ozar's discussion of conscientious refusal. For what reasons might Nurse Munson feel the need to refuse to continue caring for Mrs. Brumley? What conflicts of personal and professional values might she be experiencing? Refer to the Code for Nurses (Appendix) and other relevant ethical principles to develop an argument for her refusal.

3. Ozar identifies the problems and tensions between professional commitment and other personal values. If nurses do not deal with the kinds of value conflicts that Ozar describes in this chapter, how is it likely to affect their practice?

Bibliography

Bayles, M. D. (1979): A Problem of Clean Hands: Refusal to Provide Professional Services. Social Theory and Practice, 5(2):165.

Ozar, D. T. (1984). Patient Autonomy: Three Models of the Professional-Lay Relationship in Medicine. Theoretical Medicine, 5(1):61.

Ozar, D. T. (1985). Three Models of Professionalism and Professional Obligation in Dentistry. Journal of the American Dental Association, 110(2):173.

Rawls, J. (1971). A Theory of Social Justice. Boston: Harvard University Press.

Veatch, R. (1981). A Theory of Medical Ethics. New York: Basic Books.

EPILOGUE

At the beginning of this book we announced our intention: to show that the separation of professional issues from ethical issues is artificial.

Much of the book was devoted to identifying significant professional issues and to explaining why they are issues of significant ethical and professional concern. In some cases this has led us to make recommendations, but not always. At other times we were left with ambiguity, alternatives, and lack of resolution. This lack of resolution can be disturbing. Consensus is important but not always preferable to ambiguity and disagreement, if consensus-building involves suppressing significant but controversial ideas examined by free and open minds.

The authors have purposely refrained from trying to establish that nursing is or is not now a profession. Instead, we have drawn out the ethical implications of a claim that nursing is a profession. At the same time, we have tried to show what the rest of society has a right to expect from nursing, if it accepts nursing's claim to professional status.

The quest for a professional ethic appropriate to nursing must strike a balance between totally independent practice on the one extreme and having the conditions of practice absolutely determined by forces external to nursing on the other extreme. In steering a course between these two extremes it is important to recognize that the guide is ultimately the right of the patient to be respected as an autonomous human being. With that basis, nursing can develop an ethic that acknowledges the social realities of the world in which clients seek the expert help of professionals.

APPENDIX

FLORENCE NIGHTINGALE PLEDGE FOR NURSES

I solemnly pledge myself before God and in the presence of this assembly to pass my life in purity and to practice my profession faithfully.

I will abstain from whatever is deleterious and mischievous, and will not take or knowingly administer any harmful drug.

I will do all in my power to elevate the standard of my profession, and will hold in confidence all personal matters committed to my keeping, and all family affairs coming to my knowledge in the practice of my calling.

With loyalty will I endeavor to aid the physician in his work, and devote myself to the welfare of those committed to my care.

INTERNATIONAL COUNCIL OF NURSES: CODE FOR NURSES, 1973

The fundamental responsibility of the nurse is fourfold: to promote health, to prevent illness, to restore health and to alleviate suffering.

The need for nursing is universal. Inherent in nursing is respect for life, dignity and rights of man. It is unrestricted by considerations of nationality, race, creed, color, age, sex, politics or social status.

Nurses render health services to the individual, the family and the community and coordinate their services with those of related groups.

Nurses and People

The nurse's primary responsibility is to those people who require nursing care.

The nurse, in providing care, respects the beliefs, values and customs of the individual.

The nurse holds in confidence personal information and uses judgment in sharing this information.

Nurses and Practice

The nurse carries personal responsibility for nursing practice and for maintaining competence by continual learning.

The nurse maintains the highest standards of nursing care possible within the reality of a specific situation.

The nurse uses judgment in relation to individual competence when accepting and delegating responsibilities.

The nurse when acting in a professional capacity should at all times maintain standards of personal conduct that would reflect credit upon the profession.

Nurses and Society

The nurse shares with other citizens the responsibility for initiating and supporting action to meet the health and social needs of the public.

Nurses and Co-workers

The nurse sustains a cooperative relationship with co-workers in nursing and other fields.

The nurse takes appropriate action to safeguard the individual when his care is endangered by a co-worker or any other person.

Nurses and the Profession

The nurse plays the major role in determining and implementing desirable standards of nursing practice and nursing education.

The nurse is active in developing a core of professional knowledge.

The nurse, acting through the professional organization, participates in establishing and maintaining equitable social and economic working conditions in nursing.

A PATIENT'S BILL OF RIGHTS: AMERICAN HOSPITAL ASSOCIATION, 1973*

The American Hospital Association presents a Patient's Bill of Rights with the expectation that observance of these rights will contribute to more effective patient care and greater satisfaction for the patient, his physician and the hospital organization. Further, the Association presents these rights in the expectation that they will be supported by the hospital on behalf of its patients, as an integral part of the healing process. It is recognized that a personal relationship between the physician and the patient is essential for the provision of proper medical care. The traditional physician-patient relationship takes on a new dimension when care is rendered within an organizational structure. Legal precedent has established that the institution itself also has a responsibility to the patient. It is in recognition of these factors that these rights are affirmed.

1. The patient has the right to considerate and respectful care.

---

*Reprinted with the permission of the American Hospital Association, Copyright 1972.

2. The patient has the right to obtain from his physician complete current information concerning his diagnosis, treatment and prognosis in terms the patient can be reasonably expected to understand. When it is not medically advisable to give such information to the patient, the information should be made available to an appropriate person in his behalf. He has the right to know by name the physician responsible for coordinating his care.

3. The patient has the right to receive from his physician information necessary to give informed consent prior to the start of any procedure and/ or treatment. Except in emergencies, such information for informed consent should include but not necessarily be limited to the specific procedure and/ or treatment, the medically significant risks involved, and the probable duration of incapacitation. Where medically significant alternatives for care or treatment exist, or when the patient requests information concerning medical alternatives, the patient has the right to such information. The patient also has the right to know the name of the person responsible for the procedures and/or treatment.

4. The patient has the right to refuse treatment to the extent permitted by law, and to be informed of the medical consequences of his action.

5. The patient has the right to every consideration of his privacy concerning his own medical care program. Case discussion, consultation, examination, and treatment are confidential and should be conducted discreetly. Those not directly involved in his care must have the permission of the patient to be present.

6. The patient has the right to expect that all communications and records pertaining to his care should be treated as confidential.

7. The patient has the right to expect that within its capacity a hospital must make reasonable response to the request of a patient for services. The hospital must provide evaluation, service, and/or referral as indicated by the urgency of the case. When medically permissible a patient may be transferred to another facility only after he has received complete information and explanation concerning the needs for and alternatives to such a transfer. The institution to which the patient is to be transferred must first have accepted the patient for transfer.

8. The patient has the right to obtain information as to any relationship of his hospital to other heath care and educational institutions insofar as his care is concerned. The patient has the right to obtain information as to the existence of any professional relationships among individuals, by name, who are treating him.

9. The patient has the right to be advised if the hospital proposes to engage in or perform human experimentation affecting his care or treatment. The patient has the right to refuse to participate in such research projects.

10. The patient has the right to expect reasonable continuity of care. He has the right to know in advance what appointment times and physicians are available and where. The patient has the right to expect that the hospital

will provide a mechanism whereby he is informed by his physician or a delegate of the physician of the patient's continuing health care requirements following discharge.

11. The patient has the right to examine and receive an explanation of his bill regardless of source of payment.

12. The patient has the right to know what hospital rules and regulations apply to his conduct as a patient.

No catalogue of rights can guarantee for the patient the kind of treatment he has a right to expect. A hospital has many functions to perform, including the prevention and treatment of disease, the education of both health professionals and patients, and the conduct of clinical research. All these activities must be conducted with an overriding concern for the patient, and, above all, the recognition of his dignity as a human being. Success in achieving this recognition assures success in the defense of the rights of the patient.

1 CODE FOR NURSES WITH INTERPRETIVE STATEMENTS

The nurse provides services with respect for human dignity and the uniqueness of the client, unrestricted by considerations of social or economic status, personal attributes, or the nature of health problems.

1.1 Respect for Human Dignity

The fundamental principle of nursing practice is respect for the inherent dignity and worth of every client. Nurses are morally obligated to respect human existence and the individuality of all persons who are the recipients of nursing actions. Nurses therefore must take all reasonable means to protect and preserve human life when there is hope of recovery or reasonable hope of benefit from life-prolonging treatment.

Truth telling and the process of reaching informed choice underlie the exercise of self-determination, which is basic to respect for persons. Clients should be as fully involved as possible in the planning and implementation of their own health care. Clients have the moral right to determine what will be done with their own person; to be given accurate information, and all the information necessary for making informed judgments; to be assisted with weighing the benefits and burdens of options in their treatment; to accept, refuse, or terminate treatment without coercion; and to be given necessary emotional support. Each nurse has an obligation to be knowledgeable about the moral and legal rights of all clients and to protect and support those rights. In situations in which the client lacks the capacity to make a decision, a surrogate decision maker should be designated.

Individuals are interdependent members of the community. Taking into account both individual rights and the interdependence of persons in decision making, the nurse recognizes those situations in which individual rights to autonomy in health care may temporarily be overridden to preserve the life of the human community; for example, when a disaster demands triage or when an individual presents a direct danger to others. The many variables involved make it imperative that each case be considered with full awareness of the need to preserve the rights and responsibilities of clients and the demands of justice. The suspension of individual rights must always be considered a deviation to be tolerated as briefly as possible.

1.2 Status and Attributes of Clients

The need for health care is universal, transcending all national, ethnic, racial, religious, cultural, political, educational, economic, developmental, personality, role, and sexual differences. Nursing care is delivered without prejudicial behavior. Individual value systems and life-styles should be considered in the planning of health care with and for each client. Attributes of clients influence nursing practice to the extent that they represent factors the nurse must understand, consider, and respect in tailoring care to personal needs and in maintaining the individual's self-respect and dignity.

1.3 The Nature of Health Problems

The nurse's respect for the worth and dignity of the individual human being applies, irrespective of the nature of the health problem. It is reflected in care given the person who is disabled as well as one without disability, the person with long-term illness as well as one with acute illness, the recovering patient as well as one in the last phase of life. This respect extends to all who require the services of the nurse for the promotion of health, the prevention of illness, the restoration of health, the alleviation of suffering, and the provision of supportive care of the dying. The nurse does not act deliberately to terminate the life of any person.

The nurse's concern for human dignity and for the provision of high quality nursing care is not limited by personal attitudes or beliefs. If ethically opposed to interventions in a particular case because of the procedures to be used, the nurse is justified in refusing to participate. Such refusal should be made known in advance and in time for other appropriate arrangements to be made for the client's nursing care. If the nurse becomes involved in such a case and the client's life is in jeopardy, the nurse is obliged to provide for the client's safety, to avoid abandonment, and to withdraw only when assured that alternative sources of nursing care are available to the client.

The measures nurses take to care for the dying client and the client's family emphasize human contact. They enable the client to live with as much physical, emotional, and spiritual comfort as possible, and they maximize the values the client has treasured in life. Nursing care is directed toward the prevention and relief of the suffering commonly associated with the dying process. The nurse may provide interventions to relieve symptoms in the dying client even when the interventions entail substantial risks of hastening death.

1.4 The Setting for Health Care

The nurse adheres to the principle of nondiscriminatory, nonprejudicial care in every situation and endeavors to promote its acceptance by others. The setting shall not determine the nurse's readiness to respect clients and to render or obtain needed services.

2

The nurse safeguards the client's right to privacy by judiciously protecting information of a confidential nature.

2.1 The Client's Right to Privacy

The right to privacy is an inalienable human right. The client trusts the nurse to hold all information in confidence. This trust could be destroyed and the client's welfare jeopardized by injudicious disclosure of information provided in confidence. The duty of confidentiality, however, is not absolute when innocent parties are in direct jeopardy.

2.2 Protection of Information

The rights, well-being, and safety of the individual client should be the determining factors in arriving at any professional judgment concerning the disposition of confidential information received from the client relevant to his or her treatment. The standards of nursing practice and the nursing responsibility to provide high quality health services require that relevant data be shared with members of the health team. Only information pertinent to a client's treatment and welfare is disclosed, and it is disclosed only to those directly concerned with the client's care.

Information documenting the appropriateness, necessity, and quality of care required for the purposes of peer review, third-party payment, and other quality assurance mechanisms must be disclosed only under defined policies, mandates, or protocols. These written guidelines must assure that the rights, well-being, and safety of the client are maintained.

2.3 Access to Records

If in the course of providing care there is a need for the nurse to have access to the records of persons not under the nurse's care, the persons affected should be notified and, whenever possible, permission should be obtained first. Although records belong to the agency where the data are collected, the individual maintains the right of control over the information in the record. Similarly, professionals may exercise the right of control over information they have generated in the course of health care.

If the nurse wishes to use a client's treatment record for research or nonclinical purposes in which anonymity cannot be guaranteed, the client's consent must be obtained first. Ethically, this ensures the client's right to privacy; legally, it protects the client against unlawful invasion of privacy.

3

The nurse acts to safeguard the client and the public when health care and safety are affected by incompetent, unethical, or illegal practice by any person.

3.1 Safeguarding the Health and Safety of the Client

The nurse's primary commitment is to the health, welfare, and safety of the client. As an advocate for the client, the nurse must be alert to and take appropriate action regarding any instances of incompetent, unethical, or illegal practice by any member of the health care team or the health care system, or any action on the part of others that places the rights or best interests of the client in jeopardy. To function effectively in this role, nurses must be aware of the employing institution's policies and procedures, nursing standards of practice, the Code for Nurses, and laws governing nursing and health care practice with regard to incompetent, unethical, or illegal practice.

3.2 Acting on Questionable Practice

When the nurse is aware of inappropriate or questionable practice in the provision of health care, concern should be expressed to the person carrying out the questionable practice and attention called to the possible detrimental effect upon the client's welfare. When factors in the health care delivery system threaten the welfare of the client, similar action should be directed to the responsible administrative person. If indicated, the practice should then be reported to the appropriate authority within the institution, agency, or larger system.

There should be an established process for the reporting and handling of incompetent, unethical, or illegal practice within the employment setting so that such reporting can go through official channels without causing fear of reprisal. The nurse should be knowledgeable about the process and be prepared to use it if necessary. When questions are raised about the practices of individual practitioners or of health care systems, written documentation of the observed practices or behaviors must be available to the appropriate authorities. State nurses' associations should be prepared to provide assistance and support in the development and evaluation of such processes and in reporting procedures.

When incompetent, unethical, or illegal practice on the part of anyone concerned with the client's care is not corrected within the employment setting and continues to jeopardize the client's welfare and safety, the problem should be reported to other appropriate authorities such as practice committees of the pertinent professional organizations or the legally constituted bodies concerned with licensing of specific categories of health workers or professional practitioners. Some situations may warrant the concern and involvement of all such groups. Accurate reporting and documentation undergird all actions.

3.3 Review Mechanisms

The nurse should participate in the planning, establishment, implementation, and evaluation of review mechanisms that serve to safeguard clients, such as duly constituted peer review processes or committees and ethics committees. Such ongoing review mechanisms are based on established criteria, have stated purposes, include a process for making recommendations, and facilitate improved delivery of nursing and other health services to clients wherever nursing services are provided.

4

The nurse assumes responsibility and accountability for individual nursing judgments and actions.

4.1 Acceptance of Responsibility and Accountability

The recipients of professional nursing services are entitled to high quality nursing care.

Individual professional licensure is the protective mechanism legislated by the public to ensure the basic and minimum competencies of the professional nurse. Beyond that, society has accorded to the nursing profession the right to regulate its own practice. The regulation and control of nursing practice by nurses demand that individual practitioners of professional nursing must bear primary responsibility for the nursing care clients receive and must be individually accountable for their own practice.

4.2 Responsibility for Nursing Judgment and Action

Responsibility refers to the carrying out of duties associated with a particular role assumed by the nurse. Nursing obligations are reflected in the ANA publications *Nursing: A Social Policy Statement* and *Standards of Nursing Practice.* In recognizing the rights of clients, the standards describe a collaborative relationship between the nurse and the client through use of the nursing process. Nursing responsibilities include data collection and assessment of the health status of the client; formation of nursing diagnoses derived from client assessment; development of a nursing care plan that is directed toward designated goals, assists the client in maximizing his or her health capabilities, and provides for the client's participation in promoting, maintaining, and restoring his or her health; evaluation of the effectiveness of nursing care in achieving goals as determined by the client and the nurse; and subsequent reassessment and revision of the nursing care plan as warranted. In the process of assuming these responsibilities, the nurse is held accountable for them.

4.3 Accountability for Nursing Judgment and Action

Accountability refers to being answerable to someone for something one has done. It means providing an explanation or rationale to oneself, to clients, to peers, to the nursing profession, and to society. In order to be accountable, nurses act under a code of ethical conduct that is grounded in the moral principles of fidelity and respect for the dignity, worth, and self-determination of clients.

The nursing profession continues to develop ways to clarify nursing's accountability to society. The contract between the profession and society is made explicit through such mechanisms as (a) the Code for Nurses, (b) the standards of nursing practice, (c) the development of nursing theory derived from nursing research in order to guide nursing actions, (d) educational requirements for practice, (e) certification, and (f) mechanisms for evaluating the effectiveness of the nurse's performance of nursing responsibilities.

Nurses are accountable for judgments made and actions taken in the course of nursing practice. Neither physicians' orders nor the employing agency's policies relieve the nurse of accountability for actions taken and judgments made.

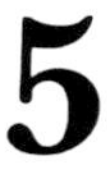

The nurse maintains competence in nursing.

5.1 Personal Responsibility for Competence

The profession of nursing is obligated to provide adequate and competent nursing care. Therefore it is the personal responsibility of each nurse to maintain competency in practice. For the client's optimum well-being and for the nurse's own professional development, the care of the client reflects and incorporates new techniques and knowledge in health care as these develop, especially as they relate to the nurse's particular field of practice. The nurse must be aware of the need for continued professional learning and must assume personal responsibility for currency of knowledge and skills.

5.2 Measurement of Competence in Nursing Practice

Evaluation of one's performance by peers is a hallmark of professionalism and a method by which the profession is held accountable to society. Nurses must be willing to have their practice reviewed and evaluated by their peers. Guidelines for evaluating the scope of practice and the appropriateness, effectiveness, and efficiency of nursing practice are found in nursing practice acts, ANA standards of practice, and other quality assurance mechanisms. Each nurse is responsible for participating in the development of objective criteria for evaluation. In addition, the nurse engages in ongoing self-evaluation of clinical competency, decision-making abilities, and professional judgments.

5.3 Intraprofessional Responsibility for Competence in Nursing Care

Nurses share responsibility for high quality nursing care. Nurses are required to have knowledge relevant to the current scope of nursing practice, changing issues and concerns, and ethical concepts and principles. Since individual competencies vary, nurses refer clients to and consult with other nurses with expertise and recognized competencies in various fields of practice.

6

The nurse exercises informed judgment and uses individual competency and qualifications as criteria in seeking consultation, accepting responsibilities, and delegating nursing activities.

6.1 Changing Functions

Nurses are faced with decisions in the context of the increased complexity of health care, changing patterns in the delivery of health services, and the development of evolving nursing practice in response to the health needs of clients. As the scope of nursing practice changes, the nurse must exercise judgment in accepting responsibilities, seeking consultation, and assigning responsibilities to others who carry out nursing care.

6.2 Accepting Responsibilities

The nurse must not engage in practices prohibited by law or delegate to others activities prohibited by practice acts of other health care personnel or by other laws. Nurses determine the scope of their practice in light of their education, knowledge, competency, and extent of experience. If the nurse concludes that he or she lacks competence or is inadequately prepared to carry out a specific function, the nurse has the responsibility to refuse that work and to seek alternative sources of care based on concern for the client's welfare. In that refusal, both the client and the nurse are protected. Inasmuch as the nurse is responsible for the continuous care of patients in health care settings, the nurse is frequently called upon to carry out components of care delegated by other health professionals as part of the client's treatment regimen. The nurse should not accept these interdependent functions if they are so extensive as to prevent the nurse from fulfilling the responsibility to provide appropriate nursing care to clients.

6.3 Consultation and Collaboration

The provision of health and illness care to clients is a complex process that requires a wide range of knowledge, skills, and collaborative efforts. Nurses must be aware of their own individual competencies. When the needs of the client are beyond the qualifications and competencies of the nurse, consultation and collaboration must be sought from qualified nurses, other health professionals, or other appropriate sources. Participation on intradisciplinary or interdisciplinary teams is often an effective approach to the provision of high quality total health services.

6.4 Delegation of Nursing Activities

Inasmuch as the nurse is accountable for the quality of nursing care rendered to clients, nurses are accountable for the delegation of nursing care activities to other health workers. Therefore, the nurse must assess individual competency in assigning selected components of nursing care to other nursing service personnel. The nurse should not delegate to any member of the nursing team a function for which that person is not prepared or qualified. Employer policies or directives do not relieve the nurse of accountability for making judgments about the delegation of nursing care activities.

7

The nurse participates in activities that contribute to the ongoing development of the profession's body of knowledge.

7.1 The Nurse and Development of Knowledge

Every profession must engage in scholarly inquiry to identify, verify, and continually enlarge the body of knowledge that forms the foundation for its practice. A unique body of verified knowledge provides both framework and direction for the profession in all of its activities and for the practitioner in the provision of nursing care. The accrual of scientific and humanistic knowledge promotes the advancement of practice and the well-being of the profession's clients. Ongoing scholarly activity such as research and the development of theory is indispensable to the full discharge of a profession's obligations to society. Each nurse has a role in this area of professional activity, whether as an investigator in furthering knowledge, as a participant in research, or as a user of theoretical and empirical knowledge.

7.2 Protection of Rights of Human Participants in Research

Individual rights valued by society and by the nursing profession that have particular application in research include the right of adequately informed consent, the right to freedom from risk of injury, and the right of privacy and preservation of dignity. Inherent in these rights is respect for each individual's rights to exercise self-determination, to choose to participate or not, to have full information, and to terminate participation in research without penalty.

It is the duty of the nurse functioning in any research role to maintain vigilance in protecting the life, health, and privacy of human subjects from both anticipated and unanticipated risks and in assuring informed consent. Subjects' integrity, privacy, and rights must be especially safeguarded if the subjects are unable to protect themselves because of incapacity or because they are in a dependent relationship to the investigator. The investigation should be discontinued if its continuance might be harmful to the subject.

7.3 General Guidelines for Participating in Research

Before participating in research conducted by others, the nurse has an obligation to (a) obtain information about the intent and the nature of the research and (b) ascertain that the study proposal is approved by the appropriate bodies, such as institutional review boards.

Research should be conducted and directed by qualified persons. The nurse who participates in research in any capacity should be fully informed about both the nurse's and the client's rights and obligations.

The nurse participates in the profession's efforts to implement and improve standards of nursing.

8.1 Responsibility to the Public for Standards

Nursing is responsible and accountable for admitting to the profession only those individuals who have demonstrated the knowledge, skills, and commitment considered essential to professional practice. Nurse educators have a major responsibility for ensuring that these competencies and a demonstrated commitment to professional practice have been achieved before the entry of an individual into the practice of professional nursing.

Established standards and guidelines for nursing practice provide guidance for the delivery of professional nursing care and are a means for evaluating care received by the public. The nurse has a personal responsibility and commitment to clients for implementation and maintenance of optimal standards of nursing practice.

8.2 Responsibility to the Profession for Standards

Established standards reflect the practice of nursing grounded in ethical commitments and a body of knowledge. Professional standards or guidelines exist in nursing practice, nursing service, nursing education, and nursing research. The nurse has the responsibility to monitor these standards in daily practice and to participate actively in the profession's ongoing efforts to foster optimal standards of practice at the local, regional, state, and national levels of the health care system.

Nurse educators have the additional responsibility to maintain optimal standards of nursing practice and education in nursing education programs and in any other settings where planned learning activities for nursing students take place.

9

The nurse participates in the profession's efforts to establish and maintain conditions of employment conducive to high quality nursing care.

9.1 Responsibility for Conditions of Employment

The nurse must be concerned with conditions of employment that (a) enable the nurse to practice in accordance with the standards of nursing practice and (b) provide a care environment that meets the standards of nursing service. The provision of high quality nursing care is the responsibility of both the individual nurse and the nursing profession. Professional autonomy and self-regulation in the control of conditions of practice are necessary for implementing nursing standards.

9.2 Maintaining Conditions for High Quality Nursing Care

Articulation and control of nursing practice can be accomplished through individual agreement and collective action. A nurse may enter into an agreement with individuals or organizations to provide health care. Nurses may participate in collective action such as collective bargaining through their state nurses' association to determine the terms and conditions of employment conducive to high quality nursing care. Such agreements should be consistent with the profession's standards of practice, the state law regulating nursing practice, and the Code for Nurses.

10

The nurse participates in the profession's effort to protect the public from misinformation and misrepresentation and to maintain the integrity of nursing.

10.1 Protection from Misinformation and Misrepresentation

Nurses are responsible for advising clients against the use of products that endanger the clients' safety and welfare. The nurse shall not use any form of public or professional communication to make claims that are false, fraudulent, misleading, deceptive, or unfair.

The nurse does not give or imply endorsement to advertising, promotion, or sale of commercial products or services in a manner that may be interpreted as reflecting the opinion or judgment of the profession as a whole. The nurse may use knowledge of specific services or products in advising an individual client, since this may contribute to the client's health and well-being. In the course of providing information or education to clients or other practitioners about commercial products or services, however, a variety of similar products or services should be offered or described so the client or practitioner can make an informed choice.

10.2 Maintaining the Integrity of Nursing

The use of the title *registered nurse* is granted by state governments for the protection of the public. Use of that title carries with it the responsibility to act in the public interest. The nurse may use the title *R.N.* and symbols of academic degrees or other earned or honorary professional symbols of recognition in all ways that are legal and appropriate. The title and other symbols of the profession should not be used, however, for benefits unrelated to nursing practice or the profession, or used by those who may seek to exploit them for other purposes.

Nurses should refrain from casting a vote in any deliberations involving health care services or facilities where the nurse has business or other interests that could be construed as a conflict of interest.

11

The nurse collaborates with members of the health professions and other citizens in promoting community and national efforts to meet the health needs of the public.

11.1 Collaboration with Others to Meet Health Needs

The availability and accessibility of high quality health services to all people require collaborative planning at the local, state, national, and international levels that respects the interdependence of health professionals and clients in health care systems. Nursing care is an integral part of high quality health care, and nurses have an obligation to promote equitable access to nursing and health care for all people.

11.2 Responsibility to the Public

The nursing profession is committed to promoting the welfare and safety of all people. The goals and values of nursing are essential to effective delivery of health services. For the benefit of the individual client and the public at large, nursing's goals and commitments need adequate representation. Nurses should ensure this representation by active participation in decision making in institutional and political arenas to assure a just distribution of health care and nursing resources.

11.3 Relationships with Other Disciplines

The complexity of health care delivery systems requires a multidisciplinary approach to delivery of services that has the strong support and active participation of all the health professions. Nurses should actively promote the collaborative planning required to ensure the availability and accessibility of high quality health services to all persons whose health needs are unmet.

INDEX